SLEEP SMARTER

21 ESSENTIAL STRATEGIES TO SLEEP YOUR WAY TO A BETTER BODY, BETTER HEALTH, AND BIGGER SUCCESS

SHAWN STEVENSON

RODALE.

RODALE *wellness*

Live happy. Be healthy. Get inspired.

Sign up today to get exclusive access to our authors, exclusive
bonuses, and the most authoritative, useful, and cutting-edge
information on health, wellness, fitness, and living your life to
the fullest.

Visit us online at RodaleWellness.com
Join us at RodaleWellness.com/Join

Portions of this book were previously published by Model House Publishing in 2014.

Rodale books may be purchased for business or promotional use or for special sales.
For information, please write to: Special Markets Department, Rodale Inc., 733 Third Avenue,
New York, NY 10017.

Printed in the United States of America
Rodale Inc. makes every effort to use acid-free ∞, recycled paper ♻.

Book design by Amy C. King

Illustrations by Paul Girard
Cartoon on page 107 reprinted with permission from Scott Metzger.

Library of Congress Cataloging-in-Publication Data is on file with the publisher.
ISBN-13: 978–1–62336–739–8

Distributed to the trade by Macmillan
2   4   6   8   10   9   7   5   3   1   hardcover

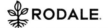

We inspire and enable people to improve their lives and the world around them.
rodalebooks.com

I still remember the feeling when my grandmother put me to sleep at night. I felt happy, I felt loved, and I felt excited about what the next day would bring. This book is dedicated to her. I will never stop representing her and sharing all of the incredible gifts that she saw in me.

It's my sincerest wish that you not only get the best sleep possible, but that your life is happier, healthier, and full of success because of it.

Contents

FOREWORD

Sleep suffers from a PR problem and desperately needs rebranding. Sleep isn't sexy. Sleep is a necessary part of life, though most of us scrape by with as little as possible. Most physicians and public health officials ignore it as a cornerstone of optimal health. Sleep just seems like a no-brainer, so few people have paid attention. Until now.

It turns out that sleep can make or break your ability to lose weight, age slowly, prevent cancer, and perform at a high level. That's because sleep regulates most hormone production. Sleep is part of your circadian rhythm, meaning that it occurs under a repeatable, 24-hour process and is determined by the light-dark cycle of your environment. At least 15 percent of your DNA is controlled by circadian rhythm, including your body's repair mechanisms.

You may be saying to yourself, "That's fine, Dr. Sara—I'll just take an Ambien and call you in the morning." Sadly, pharmaceuticals aren't the answer. Taking sleeping medication, even as little as one pill 20 times per year, has been shown in three large studies to be associated with increased mortality. Plus, your favorite prescription sleepers add only about 30 to 40 minutes of sleep to your schedule, and not necessarily high-quality sleep. Put another way, popping a prescription isn't the solution because poor sleep isn't usually from a single cause.

We need a broader-based solution. That's where Shawn Stevenson comes in.

I first met Shawn about 2 years ago, when he was a guest on my podcast. Hearing his voice, I secretly wondered how a health expert could be so cool. I tried to categorize him as a nutritionist or a trainer, but he didn't fit the mold. I listened to him tell his dramatic story of growing up in some of the harshest conditions for any child, and his story of transformation as a teenager stunned me and made me want to know more.

You see, Shawn rose above the despair of inner-city life as a scholar athlete with a lot of promise. Little did he know that his ticket out would get shut down early. He was in track practice performing a 200-meter time trial with his coach, and as he came off the curve into the straightaway, he broke his hip. Not from trauma or a fall, simply from running all out. It wasn't until years later, when he was 20, that he finally got the correct diagnosis of degenerative bone and disc disease. He had two herniated discs at L4 and L5/S1. Doctors told him: Stop competing as an athlete. Nothing can be done. Take these medications for the rest of your life.

That was a defining moment, because Shawn decided that the message from conventional medicine wasn't good enough. So he took on his diagnoses with the tenacity and focus of a sprinter and figured out on his own key principles of functional medicine: that your body cannot create and regenerate tissues if it doesn't have the necessary raw materials, and that you cannot turn over your power to a well-meaning health professional who offers no hope. In functional medicine (the type of systems-based medical care that I provide where we address the root cause of symptoms), we call it a pleiotropic solution—an approach that addresses nutrition, exercise, stress response, relationships, and self-care.

He began upgrading to organic food and increasing micronutrient density. He didn't like vegetables, so he started juicing to sneak in the benefits. And perhaps most important, he upgraded his sleep. Six weeks later, he had lost 28 pounds. His acne cleared up along with his chronic joint pain. His energy was unprecedented. Nine months later, his physician stared at his MRI scan in disbelief: Shawn's two herniated discs had healed, and he had regained lubrication in his discs. He even grew a half-inch taller. He completely reversed the degeneration.

Shawn learned that we have to take it upon ourselves to make the first steps in achieving the health we want. And he's on a mission to show you how.

Sleep is when growth hormone is released, so that your body can maintain and repair muscle and decrease belly fat. Sleep helps to consolidate your memory and literally changes the cellular structure of the brain by providing a wash of cerebral spinal fluid that removes the damaging molecules associated with neurodegeneration.

When your sleep suffers, you suffer major consequences beyond the dark circles under your eyes. You're probably grouchy and not fun to be around. Key relationships and parenting suffer. Work productivity declines. Your level of cortisol, a key stress hormone, is higher—and that makes you eat more and store belly fat. Your thyroid slows down. Insulin doesn't work as well, and your blood sugar gets out of whack. You can't clear the gunk out of your brain or soul. Your risk of cancer is quadrupled depending on the duration and volume of your sleep debt. You increase your risk of diabetes, metabolic syndrome, and heart disease.

When you improve your sleep by using the tips in this book, you'll likely experience the following benefits:

- Better skin health and a more youthful appearance
- Emotional regeneration and better relationships
- Decreased risk of stroke and cardiovascular disease
- Fewer accidents
- Lower levels of inflammation
- Enhanced function of the immune system and lower risk of cancer and infection
- Hormonal balance
- Faster rate of weight loss
- Decreased pain
- Stronger bones
- Lower risk of Alzheimer's disease and cognitive decline; better memory
- Longevity

I urge you to upgrade your sleep with Shawn Stevenson. I consider Shawn a good friend and colleague, and I know he's part cool, straight-shooting motivator and part academic. That combination makes him uniquely qualified as a new, fresh, and vital voice in the crowded space of wellness and health. Shawn knows the importance of health more than most because he hasn't always been on the receiving end of it. He's gritty and real. He wants you to find the best solutions, no matter the prognosis, because he knows from experience how to beat any prognosis. So upgrade your sleep, and you'll upgrade your health and your life.

Sara Gottfried, MD
Berkeley, California

AUTHOR'S PREFACE

Being good at sleep isn't like being good at baseball or public speaking. You don't win any awards for being a good sleeper, and no one praises you for how awesome you may be at it. Being a good sleeper is something that's generally very private—until not being a good sleeper starts to leak its way into other areas of your life.

My struggle with sleep paraded around town in a public affair with my weight and health issues, yet in many ways it was still ignored. Everyone could see the extra weight I was carrying, and they could see that I was in pain from a tremendous health problem, but no one saw the struggle I had on my pillow each night. It was a quiet suffering that I battled alone. But luckily there was light at the end of the tunnel.

I could not have found my road back to health without first paving a way to better sleep. It seems surreal sometimes that countless people around the world are sleeping better at night because of what I went through. Though there have been some extremely rough times, I wouldn't trade my experiences for the world. I've learned over time that great teachers come before us to give us the gift of accelerated growth. They struggle and find the way so that we don't have to.

We all have a story, and my story is much bigger than just finding a way to be good at sleep. As you'll discover in this book, our sleep quality (or lack thereof) is heavily influenced by our diet, exercise, stress levels, and many other pertinent lifestyle factors. For me, like everyone else, my blueprint in these areas was set at a very young age. I hope that by hearing my story, and putting what I learned into action for yourself, it leads you to the most incredible health—and sleep—that you've ever dreamed possible.

SETTING THE BAR

My mother was really young when she had me, so for the first 6 years of my life, I lived with my grandmother. She set the template for unconditional love, learning, and self-confidence. But she also set a template for my eating habits that would last for decades.

Though my grandfather would hunt and fish, and my grandmother grew food in her garden, because she wanted me to be happy and always "clean my plate," she would give me things like fish sticks, macaroni and cheese, SpaghettiOs, sandwiches, and potato chips most of the time. Occasionally I'd accept some broccoli (but only if it had a little cheese on it!). Any "weird foods" I didn't like (aka anything that didn't come in a box), she would let me slip by without eating. I know she loved me dearly, but my palate was now set for an early date with disease.

I moved in with my mom in the inner city around age 7 and carried those same habits, but my mom and stepfather would try to force me to eat—yelling, threatening, all things that naturally are going to create an even stronger apprehension of trying new foods.

Now I had even more access to foods I didn't get to see as much with my grandmother, such as fast food and candy. It was like a dream come true. I could go to the corner store and buy "penny candy" with the little pocket change I would find. I could literally get 100 pieces of candy for a dollar! I felt like I was the wealthiest kid on earth. I was swimming in candy like Scrooge McDuck swimming in his money.

I got fast food occasionally with my grandmother, but it was everywhere around me now. It was cheap enough that we could afford it, and the convenience was a huge player because my mom and stepfather worked hard, long hours to make sure we were fine.

By my first couple of years in elementary school, I had learned a lot from both environments. From my mom I learned how to survive. I learned how to make something out of nothing. I learned that no matter what happened the day before, you get up, go to work, and handle your responsibilities.

What I received from my grandmother really came in powerfully in other areas. I really understood the value of learning and was pretty passionate about listening to the wisdom of my teachers. I received numerous academic awards all through school, and I saw the real downside of drugs and alcohol in the community that I was a part of when I moved in with my mom (especially within my own home, seeing what it did to my family). It gave me a clear picture of what I *didn't* want, and my life became about making a way to live a healthy life on my terms (even though I didn't know what health really was, I knew very clearly what it wasn't).

My efforts to steer clear of drugs and alcohol and to be a high performer in school were going well. But my food decisions and daily lack of good nutrition were starting to take their toll. The first warning sign was when I was 15 years old. I was a two-sport athlete performing at a high level. Having already ran a 4.5-second 40-yard dash before the football season, I was now ready for track season to begin to really see what I could do . . . but fate had other plans.

One day at track practice, while doing a 200-meter time trial with my coach—just me and my coach on the track—as I was coming off of the curve onto the straightaway, *I broke my hip.*

No trauma, no fall, this was simply from running. I didn't know what was happening. I thought maybe I had just torn a muscle, but when I went to the physical therapist and he took an x-ray, there it was floating off in space. I pulled a muscle, and along with it came part of my iliac crest (the top of my hip bone).

I went through the standard of care: ultrasound, staying off the leg, and taking some NSAIDS (anti-inflammatory drugs). It was cool because I got to walk around with crutches and get out of class early for a few weeks. But no one ever stopped to ask: How did this 15-year-old kid's hip break? This type of thing is usually reserved for people much older. It's not the case that elderly people tend to fall and break their hips; it's that they tend to break their hips and then fall. How could this happen to me?

Fast-forward through about a dozen small injuries after that, and I was finally diagnosed with degenerative bone disease and degenerative disc disease at 20 years old. No cure. No hope for getting any better (according to my well-meaning physicians).

The very first physician who ordered an MRI put the scans of my spine up for me to see and told me what the diagnosis was. I optimistically said, "How do we fix this?"

He looked at me with a little bit of pity and said, "Son, this is incurable. You have the spine of an 80-year-old. There's nothing that you can do about it. We are going to get you some medication to manage this, but this is something you're just going to have to live with. I'm sorry."

Deflated and confused, I left the doctor's office and proceeded to get worse and worse over the following days, weeks, and months.

This was definitely the darkest spot in my life. I was in college and had to keep dropping classes because it was just too difficult to get around. I was fine once I was up walking around for a while, but every time I would sit down or lie down, in order for me to stand up again, I had to deal with what could be best described as an electric shock shooting down my leg. It was powerful enough that it would make me physically jerk. It was embarrassing and painful, and it put me in fear of even standing up.

Two and a half years went by, and I gained about 50 pounds. Following the doctor's orders of bed rest and minimal activity, I just continued to pile on the weight, eat my standard college diet, and stay up late playing Madden football video games. (Side note here: I became *awesome* at Madden.)

I continued to bank on the next physician I spoke with to give me hope, but that hope never came. It was all the same thing: Medication, bed rest, and I'm sorry that this happened. Then one night, everything changed. . . .

SECOND CHANCE

I sat on the edge of my bed in my one-bedroom college apartment with my medication bottle in my hand. I took this particular medication every night to make sure I stayed asleep, because even if I moved around in bed, the pain could be enough to wake me up.

I stared at the pill bottle, and my grandmother came rushing into my mind. . . .

She always told me how special I was. She told everyone that I would do great things, as did my mom. They believed in me. And here I was having lost belief in myself.

In that moment I realized that I'd been putting all of my hope into my doctors alone. Though they meant well, they don't walk in my shoes, and they can never have the final say about what I'm capable of.

In that moment my life changed. In that moment I made the *decision* to get well, which most people never actually do. Most of the time we hope, wish, or *try* for things to get better. Even when we pray, it's without the most important faculty of bringing that prayer to life, which is *belief.*

The word *decision* is from the Latin *de*, meaning from, and *cider*, which means to cut. So when you make a *real* decision about something, you cut away the possibility of anything happening except that thing. There is no other option except the thing that you decide upon. Come what may, you're going to have, do, and be whatever it takes to make your vision a reality. And my vision was health.

TURNING THE CORNER

I'm a very analytical person by nature. I want to know *how* something works, not solely rely on the fact that it does. I didn't just bank on my new-found decision and inspiration. I put a plan together that entailed three specific things.

For some strange reason, I asked the doctor who gave me the original diagnosis if this condition had anything to do with what I was eating, or if exercising a different way would help. He looked at me like I was from another planet and said, "This has absolutely *nothing* to do with what you're eating. And exercise isn't going to help this." He then wrote me a prescription to eat some pills. And that never did sit right with me.

If I was swallowing those pills every day, of course what I was putting in my mouth mattered! Everything that goes in my body does!

So, with this hunch, I decided to change the way I was eating. As you can imagine, my palate was now set heavily for doughnuts and pizza, so this was not a walk in the park. I had to make it easy, so I just did what I knew I could do: I stopped eating fast food and started making those foods myself (and simply upgrading the quality of my ingredients).

Instead of burgers, fries, and soda from a fast-food place, I began buying grass-fed beef and organic oven fries and throwing in a veggie that I'd actually eat on the side (usually broccoli sans cheese). Instead of soda and milk-shakes, I was drinking water like I was getting paid for it.

I noticed a significant change from small switches like that. Less inflammation, more energy, and the scale even dropping in a direction that I hadn't seen in years.

Switches like this help because conventionally raised cattle eating a diet of grains, corn, and soy are proven to have higher levels of omega-6 (pro-inflammatory) fatty acids in their tissues and less omega-3 (anti-inflammatory) fatty acids. In study after study they are also shown to have higher levels of disease, and this is where the common practice of adding antibiotics to the feed takes place, not to mention the addition of hormones to increase the yield of dairy or meat.

Does that sound normal?

Cows are ruminant animals that have evolved over millennia to eat grass. Grass is cow's food. Sure, they can eat a little of other stuff, but as soon as that ratio of natural to unnatural food gets skewed, cows start expressing diseases just like we do. And then we turn around and consume the products from these animals. You can start to see why this could be problematic. So it's important to remember: It's not just "you are what you eat." It's also, *you are what you eat ate.*

I researched like a madman and looked into what my bones and the discs in my spine were actually made of and what it took for them to be healthy. I started studying health instead of disease, and I was shocked at what I found. Things like sulfur-bearing amino acids, polysaccharides, magnesium, silica, and even vitamin C were critical to my tissue health. I wasn't getting any of those things on my fast food–based diet. The closest I came was some fancy pasteurized orange juice and milk that was "fortified" with vitamin C or calcium. That means they were added back to it in a synthetic form because the high heat processing destroys a lot of the nutrients that would normally be in it.

After upgrading the quality of my ingredients, I found out what foods I could find those nutrients in, and if I didn't like them, I started juicing them or blending them into delicious smoothies.

It's critical to understand that your body requires you to supply it with the raw materials it needs to rebuild itself. If you don't provide your body with those nutrients to regenerate those tissues, then how in the world can it do its job? I was dealing with chronic degeneration, and it was a miracle that I even made it to the age of 15 before breaking down so noticeably. I was deficient in so many things my body needed that it simply couldn't maintain my health until I changed the way I was eating. But food wasn't the only thing I needed to change.

BRINGING IT ALL TOGETHER

After getting on track with my food, I started exercising again. This was nothing crazy. I just took my time and progressed each day. I started off on a stationary bike, then transitioned to walking, to a little jogging, to picking up the weights again, to eventually being able to do a lot more "normal" activities. Your body literally *requires* movement in order to heal itself. Even when we're taking in powerful nutrients through our diets (as I was now doing), our bodies increase their assimilation of these nutrients through movement.

In figuring out how this works, I came across a study done on racehorses. If a racehorse breaks a bone, it could be grounds for the animal to be put down, so there is a vested interest in improving their bone density. In this particular study, the researchers gave the horses supplements along with their normal diet and found that there was a negligible increase in their bone density. However, when the horses were *walked*, in addition to supplementation and their normal diet, the researchers noted a substantial increase in their bone density.

I got it! Real food, plus movement, equals a greatly increased shot at getting what I wanted. But there was still one missing piece. . . .

As I started to put the care and attention into my body that it had longed so much for over the years, I naturally started to get to bed earlier and get up earlier. Number one, I felt excited about life again as things were changing, and number two, my body really wanted sleep because of all of the changes it was making thanks to the exercise and good nutrition I was taking in during the day. I was beginning to realize how much sleep mattered, yet I still didn't grasp just how powerful it was until years later when I started my clinical practice.

As you'll discover, your body actually does the vast majority of healing while you're asleep. Good sleep is where I found the greatest leverage to change my health and my body. And this is what completed the three pillars of health that changed everything for me: right nutrition, right exercise, and right sleep.

Six weeks after that decision I made on the edge of my bed, I had lost 28 pounds, I had a complete transformation in my levels of energy, and, most important, the pain that I had been experiencing every single day for the last $2^1/_2$ years was gone.

I was sort of in shock. I mean, how could this be? But after going over what I had done, it all made sense. Your body really does work on a use-it-or-lose-it basis. If you put a cast on your arm, the muscles and tissues of that arm will atrophy. Well, I had put a cast on my whole body—a psychological prison where I was powerless and hardly moved. I was afraid to move.

But when I put the fear aside, implemented the things my genes had been expecting of me, and took responsibility for my body again, I broke out of the cast and didn't just get back my life—I got an even better one.

THE START OF SOMETHING SPECIAL

I was still attending my university during this time, and professors and students alike started asking me what I had done. I remember walking out of class and the teacher stopping me. He looked me right in the eyes and said, "What happened? You look so healthy!" As if an accident had occurred.

I didn't just look like a person who had lost weight. I looked like someone who was radiantly healthy. My skin glowed, my body was strong, and I walked with confidence that few people had seen before. I walked with confidence because I *could* walk—and I realized that there was always an opportunity to turn things around.

About 9 months after my initial moment of decision, I went back to my latest physician and got a scan of my spine done. He put it up and just stood looking at it with his hand on his chin for what seemed like an eternity. He turned to me and said, "Whatever you're doing, keep doing it. Things look good, my friend. I haven't seen results like this before." The two herniated discs I had (L4 and L5/S1) had retracted on their own, and some of the "juiciness" had been returned to the discs in my back.

I walked out of there with a new lease on life, and I knew that all I had gone through was for a bigger purpose.

Students, professors, and faculty at my university started asking me for help. That was really the birthing of my career. I got certified as a strength and conditioning coach and shifted as many of my remaining college courses as I could to anything and everything related to health.

Since then, I've had the opportunity to work with thousands of people in a one-on-one context, and, at this point, many hundreds of thousands of people directly through books, programs, keynotes, workshops, and my number one rated podcast, and the reach is growing every day. I have so much gratitude for what I went through, and I wouldn't change it for anything. It's the tough times that can sometimes bring out the best in us. What I went through has allowed me to be of service in the lives of so many others. Actually, gratitude isn't even a strong enough word for how I feel.

I wanted to share this story with you because there are many lessons to glean from it. First of all: *decisions*. There's a certain power to being truly committed to something. When you tap into the "Come what may! Nothing can stop me!" power that you have within you, it's amazing the changes that you can make. Whether it's improving your sleep or any other area of your life, challenges may arise, but you'll always find a way to make it through them by harnessing your power to choose.

Second: the power of nutrition, exercise, and sleep. You literally get to decide what you make your cells and tissues out of. Your decisions about what you put on your plate are not just impacting you; they are impacting every single part of you. That power is in your hands.

Exercise is not about a flat belly and six-pack abs. Sure, those things can be a part of it, but exercise is far more important than that. Exercise radically increases the assimilation of nutrients and, more important, aids in the elimination of metabolic wastes, moving your lymphatic system, and pushing toxic waste out of your body.

To take it a step further, it's really about *movement*, not just exercise. Exercise is something people tend to do for maybe an hour a day, but then what about the other 23 hours? People who exercise for an hour a day are only 4 percent more active than people who don't exercise at all. Sure, that 4 percent matters, but deciding to live a life of movement and health isn't optional today. It's something that your genes expect you to do.

Sleep is the force multiplier. It will magnify the results you get from your food and movement in the most amazing way if you allow it to. That's what this book is all about.

Within these pages you'll discover the clinically proven strategies that have helped countless people to begin getting the best sleep of their lives. You're going to find out exactly why sleep is so valuable to changing your body, your health, and even the levels of fulfillment and success in your life. Your sleep quality and the quality of your life go hand in hand. Learning to sleep smarter is going to be one of the most valuable things you'll ever do in the pursuit of living a great life on your terms. Here's to many nights of great sleep, and many days of good health and success!

Introduction

Sleep is the secret sauce.

There isn't one facet of your mental, emotional, or physical performance that's not affected by the quality of your sleep.

The big challenge is that in our fast-paced world today, millions of people are chronically sleep deprived and suffering the deleterious effects of getting low-quality sleep.

The consequences of sleep deprivation aren't pretty either. Try immune system failure, diabetes, cancer, obesity, depression, and memory loss, just to name a few. Most people don't realize that their continuous sleep problems are also a catalyst for the diseases and appearance issues they're experiencing.

Studies have shown that just one night of sleep deprivation can make you as insulin resistant as a person with type 2 diabetes. This translates directly to aging faster, decreased libido, and storing more body fat than you want to (say it ain't so!). Now stretch that out over weeks, months, even years, and you can start to see why lack of sleep can be such a huge problem.

A study published in the *Canadian Medical Association Journal* showed that sleep deprivation is directly related to an inability to lose weight. Test subjects were put on the same exercise and diet program, but those who were in the sleep deprivation group (fewer than 6 hours per night) consistently lost less weight and body fat than those in the control group, who slept for more than 8 hours per night. Could high-quality sleep be the missing component to nutrition and smart exercise to help you shed fat for good?

In Chapters 11 and 13, we'll be exploring the sleep–body fat connection and specific strategies to help you get in the best shape of your life. Pour on that secret sauce please!

Other studies show that sleep deprivation encourages cancer, Alzheimer's, depression, and even heart disease. One such study cited in the journal *Sleep* followed 98,000 people for 14 years and discovered that women who got fewer than 4 hours of sleep per night were twice as likely to die prematurely from heart disease.

In no way does that mean that the fellas are off the hook. Men are more likely to die from heart disease as it is, but add sleep deprivation to the mix and you have a real recipe for trouble. A study reported by the World Health Organization tracked the results of 657 men over a 14-year period. They found that men with poor sleep quality were also twice as likely to have a heart attack and up to 4 times more likely to have a stroke during the study period.

Heart disease is one of the biggest killers in the world today. Pulling back the veil and uncovering how sleep deprivation is a part of many of our health problems is one of the biggest steps in finding a solution.

REMEMBER THAT YOU ARE NOT ALONE

As it stands, 60 percent of people in the United States say that they have difficulties sleeping every night (or at least every other night). Sleep loss is a common condition in developed countries overall. Evidence shows that people in Western countries are sleeping on average $1\frac{1}{2}$ to 2 full hours per night less than we did just a century ago. It has become a chronic issue that somehow we have "forgotten" how to do something that should come completely naturally to us as human beings.

It took nearly a decade of clinical practice before I took a good hard look at sleep myself. Day after day I would see incredible success stories from people who implemented my nutrition and exercise advice. I was immensely grateful for that, and happy for my clients, but there was something that continued to be a virtual thorn in my side.

I couldn't seem to take my mind off of the percentage of people who seemed to do everything right but still weren't able to achieve the results that other people had. They ate an incredible diet, they exercised (oftentimes too much), yet they still couldn't seem to optimize their hormone function, balance their blood sugar levels, get the scale to budge, or whatever their main target was. Their passion and persistence was just an exercise in futility, and eventually they would fall into a place of learned helplessness or just give up altogether.

After years of being unable to crack this mystery, I finally began to do a deeper analysis and examine the daily lifestyle factors that could be coming into play.

MEAN GENES

Many people have unknowingly bought into the idea of genetic control—essentially believing that our genes control everything about us. I have genes for heart disease; I have genes for arthritis; I have some really strong fat genes that won't allow me to fit into my skinny jeans!

Even though our genes play a huge role in our health, they are in no way where the story begins or ends. There is a booming field of science called *epigenetics* that is looking at our genetic expression in a totally new way. "Epi" means above. (Thus, your "epidermis" is the layer *above* your dermis, or the outermost portion of your skin.) Epigenetics is looking at what's *above* our genetic control, and what has been discovered is fascinating.

As it turns out, our genes are not what directly control our health, appearance, and personality, as many of us once believed. Our genes are sort of like a blueprint, and within that blueprint are different options for how our structure will be built. Thousands of hours of genetic research have uncovered that we humans collectively share the same *20,000 to 25,000 genes*. That's it!

This number has been revised down drastically from the originally estimated 100,000-plus genes, and it will likely continue to drop as gene discovery methods improve. So, the question arises, if we all share the same 25,000 or fewer genes, how in the world do we have such a variation in the way we all look? In the level of health we experience? In the way that our lives turn out?

To put it simply, our environment, our lifestyle, and the decisions we make (either consciously or unconsciously) are determining which genes are getting expressed every second of our lives. We all have genes for diseases, but some people never experience them. We all have genes for optimal health and normal function, but some people struggle to ever see that as a reality.

Today we have to be empowered enough to know that we, in fact, have a huge impact on the way our health turns out. This is really nothing new if you think about it. We know that a person will likely turn out healthier if he or she doesn't smoke a pack of cigarettes every day. The physical changes that happen as a result of the person's smoking habit are a different genetic expression, and even mutation of genes, based on the decision to put that butt in their mouth every day. Yes, it is as bad as it sounds.

We also know that the food we eat can drastically change the way we look and feel. There's a whole flourishing field of science called *nutrigenomics* that's looking at the way every single bite of food you eat is impacting your genetic expression. Now stretch this understanding of epigenetics out into the realm of sleep. There may be nothing more powerful in influencing the way you look and feel than the quality of sleep you're getting.

Research published in *Current Neurology and Neuroscience Reports* found that sleep plays a huge role in the function of our DNA and RNA. The study reported that "these epigenetic mechanisms are clearly regulated by the circadian clock," encapsulating the point that your sleep is going to determine the quality of the "copies" that your body prints out of you. Sleep can determine whether your body is printing out the cells of a sexy beast or the cells of a wildebeest. We ultimately get to decide.

In my practice I started doing an analysis to help every single person uncover what epigenetic influences were hiding in plain sight. I asked them about work, I asked them about their relationships, I asked them about their habits from the time they got up in the morning to the moment they laid their head down at night. After doing this analysis, looking at blood work, and looking at hormone panels, one thing became crystal clear. All of the individuals struggling to get results had a huge problem with one of two things: sleep or stress. And most of the time it was both, as poor sleep and stress often come hand in hand.

There were dozens of stress management practices they had access to, but very few methods of improving sleep outside of the cookie-cutter advice to "sleep 8 hours." I knew this wasn't the only solution because many people got 8 hours of sleep, but they still woke up feeling exhausted and dragged around with low energy every day. This sent me on a mission to help them find ways to radically improve the *quality* of their sleep and not just the quantity. When they began to put these strategies into action, it was as if the floodgates opened, and all the results they'd been struggling to get came rushing in almost effortlessly. I was well aware of what the data showed on the importance of high-quality sleep, but to see it firsthand was life-changing.

Many of the clinically proven strategies my patients used are here in this book. And the funny thing is, at really no point did I tell them to sleep more; it was really about *sleeping smarter*. The quality of sleep they were getting was radically transformed, which led to radical transformations in their bodies, minds, and even the success in their lives.

WHAT TO EXPECT

In a society that's overworked and under-rested, it's more important than ever to pay attention to issues associated with not getting the sleep that we require. Although we'll be covering the negative impact of sleep problems in this book, we're going to put our major focus on what you can do to improve your sleep starting *tonight*, and avoid these chronic issues in the first place.

But what about performance in your work? What about productivity and getting things done?

At first glance we might think that working more and skimping on sleep will get us there faster. The research is in, and it's 100 percent conclusive: When you don't sleep well, you get slower, less creative, and more stressed, and you underperform. Basically, you're utilizing only a fraction of what you're capable of. We're going to talk about this more in Chapter 1, so sit tight and I'll give you the lowdown on what sleep (or lack thereof) is doing to your brain.

There's an old Irish proverb that says, "A good laugh and a long sleep are the two best cures for anything." My promise to you is that this book will give you real, practical strategies to help you get the best sleep possible.

You'll laugh, you'll think, you'll plan, you'll put strategies into action, and you'll see your life transformed as a result of it.

You deserve to be healthy, happy, and fulfilled in your life. Getting great sleep is a huge component of this, and this book is the key to helping you get there.

You are going to be given 21 proven strategies you can utilize to immediately improve the quality of your sleep. You can use one or all of the tips depending on your own unique goals and lifestyle. As a special bonus, at the end of the book, you'll receive a 14-Day Sleep Makeover plan to help you put everything together for the best results possible.

A pioneer and leading authority on sleep research, William Dement, MD, said, "You're not healthy, unless your sleep is healthy."

Nothing could be more true, and these 21 tips are going to help you get great sleep for many years to come.

KNOW THE VALUE OF SLEEP

The topic of this chapter is a little unusual, but it's probably the most important. Many people are negligent about getting enough sleep because they don't truly understand the benefits they could be getting from it. Once you understand the advantages of getting high-quality sleep, you'll be passionate about to putting these strategies into action for yourself.

So what is sleep? And why is it important?

Well, defining sleep is a lot like trying to define life. No one completely understands it, and if you try to explain it, you're more likely to sound like Forrest Gump than a world-renown scholar. (Life is like a box of chocolates . . . sleep is like pretending to be dead.)

The Free Dictionary defines sleep as a *natural periodic state of rest for the mind and body, in which the eyes usually close and consciousness is completely or partially lost, so that there is a decrease in bodily movement and responsiveness to external stimuli.*

That sounds a little weird, but the most important takeaway is that it's a *natural* periodic state of rest for the mind and body. If you're not doing it, then you're being completely unnatural. And nobody likes unnatural people.

What's more important is knowing the big prizes that sleep gives you.

Generally, being awake is catabolic (breaks you down) and being asleep is anabolic (builds you up). Sleep is known to be an elevated *anabolic state*, heightening the growth and rejuvenation of the immune, skeletal, and muscular systems. Basically, sleep rebuilds you and keeps you youthful.

High-quality sleep fortifies your immune system, balances your hormones, boosts your metabolism, increases your physical energy, and improves the function of your brain. Unless you give your body the right amount of sleep, you will never, I repeat *never*, have the body and life you want to have.

In our culture, sleep is not respected very much at all. In fact, we are often programmed with the idea that to be successful, we need to work harder, we need to sleep less, and we can catch up on all the sleep we want when we're dead. To say sleep is not respected is really an understatement.

Working hard is unarguably a big part of being successful, but so is working smart. So many people in our world today go on plugging away with work, burning the candle at both ends, not realizing that the *quality* of work they're doing is being radically compromised. Research shows that after just 24 hours of sleep deprivation, there is an overall reduction of 6 percent in glucose reaching the brain. Simple translation: You get dumber.

This is also why you crave candy, chips, doughnuts, and other starchy, sugary things when you're sleep deprived. Your body is trying to compel you to get that glucose back to your brain as soon as possible. It's a built-in survival mechanism. This is inherent in our genes because, in our days as hunter-gatherers, that lack of brainpower could mean a swift death from a predator or a substantially reduced ability to hunt and procure our own food for survival. Today, a simple trip to the refrigerator can bypass your body's cry for more sleep, but those stress mechanisms are still alive and well within your body right now.

I CAN'T BELIEVE I DID THAT LAST NIGHT

The most valuable takeaway from this sleep deprivation "brain drain" discovery is that the reduction in glucose isn't shared equally. Your parietal lobe and the prefrontal cortex actually lose 12 to 14 percent of their glucose when you don't sleep. These are the areas of the brain we most need for thinking, for distinguishing between ideas, for social control, and for being able to tell the difference between right and wrong. Have you ever made a poor decision when you were up late at night that you wouldn't have made if your head was on right? Chances are you have.

It wasn't entirely your fault. Your brain was hijacked by a dumber (and slightly less attractive) version of yourself.

When you're sleep deprived, you are unknowingly setting up a steel cage match between your willpower and your biology. Sure, you might be committed to eating healthier, exercising more, or even choosing better relationships. But when your prefrontal cortex starts to shut down, if you've ever had a potato chip, if you've ever had sugary cereal, if you've ever had ice cream, your brain knows that it can find a quick source of glucose in those things and shuttle it back to where it is needed. Your willpower is now in a judo-style armbar as your entire body will compel you to seek those foods out.

The next thing you know, you have cheesy fingertips from jamming down a whole bag of cheese puffs, or you find yourself looking down the barrel of an empty pint of ice cream. Upset and defeated, you blame yourself, not realizing that you were set up for failure in the first place. When you are tired, you are not yourself. Well, at least not the best version of yourself. Being sleep-deprived will automatically stack the deck against you.

By sleeping smarter, you're going to be able to stack the conditions in your favor and put healthy choices on autopilot. You're going to get a ton of tips and strategies to make that happen, but first we need to take a look at how that sleepy brain is affecting the rest of your life.

PUT IT TO THE TEST

A study published by the American Academy of Sleep Medicine found that poor sleep quality was equal to binge drinking and marijuana use in determining academic performance. The study reported that college students who were poor sleepers were much more likely to earn worse grades and even drop out of classes than their healthy sleeping peers.

Finding out that poor sleep can be as detrimental to learning as binge drinking should be a real eye-opener. Learning is a big part of our lives no matter what stage we're at. Our ability to learn and retain information is paramount to our success.

Whether we're in school or in the workforce, we'll often sacrifice sleep in the name of getting things done. But it's important to remember that there's a big difference between "working" and actually being effective.

By forgoing your sleep, you can absolutely do more work, but the quality and effectiveness of your work will be sacrificed. A study published in *The Lancet* that looked at a group of physicians proved that sleep-deprived individuals took 14 percent longer to complete a task and made 20 percent more errors than individuals who were well rested. Not only are we taking longer to do the same task, but we're going to have to spend even more time trying to go back to clean up the mess we've made.

If you learn to structure your time to get more sleep *first,* then you'll be able to get your work done faster and more effectively than if you zombie-walked your way through it. You'll be able to be more creative and energetic, and you'll have greater access to the parts of your brain responsible for problem-solving. The cultural idea of sleeping when you're dead will only accelerate the day that it becomes your reality. And the impact that sleep deprivation has on your brain will make your life a whole lot harder while you're still here to enjoy it.

YOUR BRAIN NEEDS A REHAB

Since the beginning of documented human history, philosophers and scientists alike have postulated what the real purpose of sleep is. Since it's this weird state that we're in, unconscious to the world around us, this would be the time that we'd be most vulnerable to danger and predation. From an evolutionary perspective, you'd think that we would have evolved out of sleep by now if it was making it tougher on our survival.

But what's been discovered is that sleep is actually what has enabled us to grow and evolve to the incredible level we have. Sleep hasn't been an evolutionary problem; it's been an evolutionary catalyst.

The human brain is the most powerful structure on the planet. It has enabled us to build our bodies and to build skyscrapers—to build automobiles and to build spaceships—to unlock the power of technology to create the Internet and to unlock the power of our DNA to understand life. Our brains can think externally of any new circumstance, analyze the past, forecast the future, and create limitless strategies to get there.

Billions of brain cells are controlling every function in your body as well. It's important to understand that each brain cell is capable of doing what your whole body does. These cells eat, communicate, reproduce, and even make waste. Scientists have discovered that this process of waste removal might be one of the biggest connections to our critical need for high-quality sleep.

Your body has what is essentially a cellular waste management system called the lymphatic system. It's responsible for eliminating metabolic waste and toxins to keep you healthy. However, the lymphatic system does not include your brain. This is because your brain is a closed system controlled by the blood-brain barrier, which decides what can go through and what cannot. Your brain is heavily guarded by cellular bouncers that can spot a fake ID a mile away.

Scientists have found that the brain actually has its own unique waste disposal system, similar to that of the lymphatic system. It's called the *glymphatic* system—with the added "g" as a special shout-out to the glial cells in the brain that control it.

All of the dynamic functions the human brain does result in a lot of waste products, all of which need to be removed. This waste removal literally makes room for new growth and development. Removing and recycling dead cells, tossing out toxins, and shuttling out waste is critical to brain function.

Researchers at the Center for Translational Neuromedicine at the University of Rochester Medical Center have discovered exactly how sleep relates to all of this. During sleep, the glymphatic system becomes *10 times* more active than during wakefulness. Simultaneously, your brain cells are reduced in size by about 60 percent while you're asleep to make waste removal even more efficient.

Because your brain is so active while you're awake (learning, developing, and helping you to be awesome), it's continuously building up a lot of by-products that are mainly removed by the restorative power of sleep.

If the waste removal system in your home gets backed up, then things are going to get real nasty, real fast. The same thing holds true if you're not sleeping well and your glymphatic system doesn't get to do its job. As a matter of fact, an inability of your brain to remove harmful waste products is believed to be one of the foundational causes of Alzheimer's disease.

DON'T SLEEP ON SLEEP

We've just covered a small slice of the pie on why sleep needs to be a top priority on your list from this day forward.

Always remember the value of your sleep. You will perform better, make better decisions, and have a better body when you get the sleep you require. Sleep is not an obstacle we need to go around. It's a natural state your body requires to boost your hormone function; heal your muscles, tissues, and organs; protect you from diseases; and make your mind work at its optimal level. The shortcut to success is not made by bypassing dreamland. You will work better, be more efficient, and get more stuff done when you're properly rested.

◇ ◇ ◇ ◇

SLEEP
POWER TIP #1

When you know you have a big task, project, or event coming up, pull out a calendar and plan ahead how you can get your ideal number of sleep hours in. Oftentimes it's as simple as setting up a schedule. But people overlook it because, well, it's just too easy.

If it's important to you, you'll schedule it. Stick to that schedule as well as you can, and know that you will get the work done better and faster if you're more rested. We usually sacrifice our sleep to cram in more work because we didn't plan efficiently. And as the wise Benjamin Franklin said, "By failing to prepare, you are preparing to fail."

POWER TIP #2

Begin reframing your idea of sleep. Instead of seeing sleep as an obstacle to work around (something you "have to" do), start seeing it as a special treat for yourself (something that you "get to" do) and love the entire process.

A real change begins with a simple change in your perception. Start to think of sleep as an incredible indulgence, like a sensuous dessert, a relaxing massage, a hot date with someone special, or something else that you really look forward to. "I've got a hot date with sleep tonight, and we are really going to *get—it—on!*" Start letting go of the stress surrounding sleep and allow yourself to enjoy it. You work hard enough in your life as it is. Treat yourself to some incredible sleep. You deserve it.

◇ ◇ ◇ ◇

Now that we've gotten to the deeper connection as to why your sleep is so valuable, it's time to dive into the real nuts and bolts of sleeping smarter. You're about to be equipped with some powerhouse tools and tips that you'll be able to utilize for a lifetime of great sleep. Let's go!

CHAPTER 2

GET MORE SUNLIGHT DURING THE DAY

A great night's sleep begins the moment you wake up in the morning. Humans have evolved with a predictable pattern of light and darkness that has always controlled our sleep cycles. Your sleep cycle, or *circadian timing system*, is heavily impacted by the amount of sunlight you receive during the day.

It may sound counterintuitive that getting more sunlight during the day can help you sleep better at night, but science has proven that this is precisely the case.

Your body's circadian timing system is not just some airy-fairy thing. This is a real, built-in, 24-hour clock that's not that much different from the clock on your cell phone or wristwatch. There are certain times of day that your body is designed to release specific hormones. This circadian timing system, along with the scheduled release of hormones, helps to control your digestion, immune system, blood pressure, fat utilization, appetite, and mental energy, among other things.

GENERAL CIRCADIAN RHYTHMS IN HUMANS

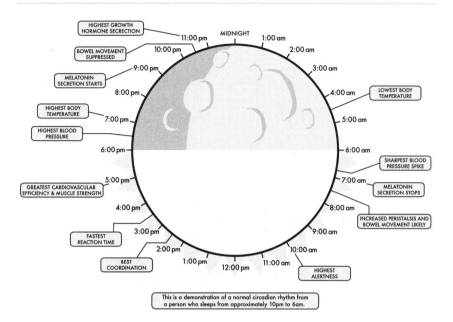

This is a demonstration of a normal circadian rhythm from a person who sleeps from approximately 10pm to 6am.

Your circadian timing system is regulated by the *suprachiasmatic nucleus*, a small group of nerve cells found in the hypothalamus in your brain. The hypothalamus is considered to be the master gland of your body's hormonal system. It controls your body's hunger, thirst, fatigue, body temperature, and sleep cycles by acting as a master clock. So, now you know, when it comes to sleep, you've literally got to have your head in the game.

Now, how does morning light improve sleep? Light actually signals your hypothalamus and all corresponding organs and glands to be alert and "wake up." That light exposure, specifically *sunlight* exposure, triggers your body to produce optimal levels of daytime hormones and neurotransmitters that regulate your biological clock. Too little light exposure during the day and too much artificial light exposure in the evening will negatively impact your ability to sleep well at night. One of the most vital compounds affected by light exposure is the powerful neurotransmitter serotonin.

THE OPENING ACT

Serotonin is commonly known to help bring about feelings of happiness and well-being. Many antidepressant drugs are centered on the function of serotonin because of its incredible effect on mood and cognition. Another important thing to note about serotonin is that it's crucial to regulating your body's internal clock.

Approximately 95 percent of your body's serotonin is located in your gastrointestinal tract, which comes as a surprise to most people. Serotonin production doesn't just magically happen on its own. It's influenced by your diet, it's influenced by your activity level, and it's also influenced by the amount of natural sunlight you get.

Our eyes have special light receptors that send information to the center of the brain (where your hypothalamus is hanging out) to trigger the production of more serotonin. This is happening day in and day out when we are living in sync with nature and our body clock is set to the right time. However, if our body clock is on the fritz, and we are not getting enough exposure to natural light, our serotonin production—and our health—is going to suffer.

In his book *The Mind-Body Mood Solution*, clinical psychologist Jeffrey Rossman, PhD, states that "many of us are not aware that we are light deprived and suffering from the effects of light deprivation. Because of our eyes' extraordinary ability to adapt to changes in brightness, we tend not to be aware of how little light we actually receive when we are indoors. Typical indoor lighting is 100 times less bright than outdoor light on a sunny day. Even a cloudy day delivers 10 times more brightness than ordinary indoor lighting."

So, how do we take action on this information when millions of us are certified desk jockeys and cooped up in our offices all day long? And how much does it matter anyway?

A recent study that focused on the sleep quality of day-shift office workers revealed some shocking results. When compared to office workers who have direct access to windows at work, those office workers who *didn't* have access to windows got 173 percent less exposure to natural light and, as a result, slept an average of 46 minutes less each night. This sleep deficit resulted in more reported physical ailments, lower vitality, and poorer sleep quality.

The office workers with more natural light exposure tended to be more physically active and happier, and they had an overall higher quality of life. Sounds like serotonin is doing its job, right? Well, this is only a small slice of the pie.

Not only is serotonin rooted in your belly, it is also located in blood platelets, your central nervous system, and even your skin.

Serotonin and serotonin transporters have been found in human keratinocytes (our predominant type of skin cell) and are heavily influenced by exposure to sunlight. Your skin absorbs UV rays from the sun that automatically promote the production of more vitamin D and serotonin. Vitamin D also has a strong link to sleep health (which we'll talk about in Chapter 7), but the role of serotonin and sleep can't be overstated enough. This is because the production of serotonin actually does set you up for a good night's sleep. According to experts at the Federation of American Societies for Experimental Biology, human skin can produce serotonin and transform it into melatonin.

MELLOW MELATONIN

Melatonin is really the star of the show when it comes to getting great sleep. Serotonin is the hype man for melatonin, getting the cellular crowd ready and getting everyone lined up for an awesome sleep performance. "Did you see that melatonin show last night? Nope. I slept right through it!"

Melatonin is produced by the pineal gland and other tissues in your body that send signals to your cells to prepare you for sleep. It's secreted naturally as it gets darker outside, but we can really screw it up if we don't get the right light exposure at the right time. Melatonin isn't really the "sleep hormone" because it doesn't directly put you to sleep. But it can definitely be considered the "get good sleep hormone" because it improves your sleep *quality* by helping to create the optimal conditions in your body for getting amazing sleep.

Some researchers believe that melatonin is related to aging. For instance, young children have the highest levels of nighttime melatonin production, but it gradually declines as we age. Melatonin is associated with being young and vital, but it diminishes as the years pass by. Is this simply how it has to be, or is it something we cause by not honoring our sleep cycles?

Even though melatonin levels naturally decline as you age, when you sleep smarter, there won't be such a dramatic drop-off, and you can sleep like a baby for more years of your life. Remember, the production and secretion of melatonin is heavily affected by light exposure. Sunlight provides the natural spectrum of light that we need to help coordinate the cycle of melatonin production. Simply put, when you get more sunlight exposure during the day, and less light exposure at night, you're on your way to a magic sleep formula that really works.

CORTISOL, THE UGLY DUCKLING

One of the other important daytime hormones that you've probably heard a lot about recently is *cortisol*. Cortisol has become a big catchword for health issues today because it's been labeled as a problematic "stress hormone." Of the more than 50 hormones the human body secretes and circulates, cortisol has been singled out as the problem child.

Cortisol is making you fat! Cortisol is causing your hormone struggles! Cortisol canceled your favorite television series! If we can do away with cortisol, everything will be all right (and we'll finally get to see David Hasselhoff back on TV).

The reality is, cortisol isn't a bad guy at all. Cortisol is incredibly important to the optimal health and performance of your body. Your body produces it for a reason. The real goal isn't to have as little cortisol as possible; it's to have a healthy rhythm of cortisol production to get you the results you want, when you want them.

This may not fit the popular description of cortisol, but it's actually somewhat of a superhero. Cortisol gives you the energy and gusto to get up and move around. It enables you to be awake and alert. It contributes to your strength, focus, and vitality every day. It's not that cortisol is bad; it's when it's being over- or underproduced that challenges can arise.

Alan Christianson, NMD, *New York Times* bestselling author and writer of *The Adrenal Reset Diet*, wonderfully states that "cortisol is an adrenal hormone that manages your body's daily rhythm. Think of it as your built-in coffeepot. You wake up in the morning because your adrenals just made a fresh batch of it. You fall asleep at night because they shut it off."

Cortisol is essential to your circadian timing system for sleep. As you can see in the chart below, you naturally have an increase in cortisol in the morning, which is for the purpose of getting up, being active, and enjoying life. Then, as you see, there is a natural reduction in cortisol as the day goes on, bottoming out in the evening to set up a great night's sleep. This is a normal cortisol rhythm, but as you know, our lives can be anything but normal.

Some of us have peaks of cortisol when it should be low, and low cortisol when it should be peaked. *Tired and wired* aptly describes this person. Physiologically you are tired at night, but you seem to be your most alert. And during the morning, when you should feel refreshed, it's almost impossible to peel your body away from the mattress. If this sounds familiar to you, then the strategies outlined in this book are going to help you transform your sleep in the most amazing way possible.

CIRCADIAN RELEASE OF CORTISOL

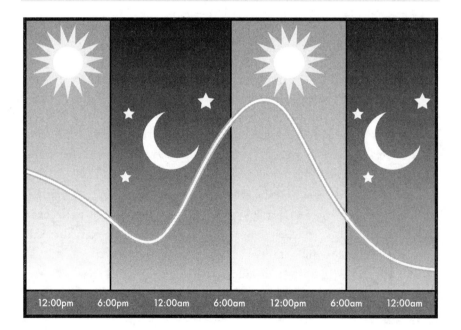

| 12:00pm | 6:00pm | 12:00am | 6:00am | 12:00pm | 6:00am | 12:00am |

One of the biggest takeaways to note is that cortisol and melatonin have somewhat of an inverse relationship. Essentially, when cortisol is up, melatonin is down. When melatonin is up, cortisol is down. Encouraging the production of the right hormone at the right time will automatically support the normal function of the other hormone.

Yet another reason why daytime exposure to sunlight is so important is that it encourages the production of cortisol. Again, this is a normal function, based on evolutionary biology, to get us up and active to procure our food, build and support our habitat, and care for our loved ones during the day. Research published in the journal *Innovations in Clinical Neuroscience* found an additional bonus: Exposure to sunlight significantly decreased cortisol levels later in the day when compared to being exposed to dim light during the day. By getting more exposure to sunlight, you set the tempo for a normal cortisol rhythm, and a normal melatonin rhythm as well.

Now that you've gained a new understanding of how sunlight affects your sleep and hormone function, it really becomes obvious how important this is. Your genes literally expect you to get exposure to sunlight in order to manage your sleep-wake cycles. But, since the world we live in is far different from the world our ancestors experienced, let's dive into how to safely and effectively leverage this to get the best results possible.

◇ ◇ ◇ ◇

SUNLIGHT
POWER TIP #1

When it comes to sleep benefits, all sunlight is not created equal. The body clock is most responsive to sunlight in the early morning, between 6:00 a.m. and 8:30 a.m. Exposure to sunlight later is still beneficial but doesn't provide the same benefit. Of course, this is going to vary depending on the time of the year, but make it a habit to get some sun exposure during that prime-time light period.

Getting direct sunlight outdoors for at least half an hour has been shown to produce the most benefit. During the winter months, it is not always feasible to get the sunlight directly on your skin. However, as you've learned, being able to take in natural light through your eyes is a part of the solution you can always utilize. Even on a cloudy day, your body will give you a favorable response.

POWER TIP #2

If you are stuck in a cubical dungeon away from natural light at work, use your break time to strategically go and get some sun on your skin. Even on an overcast day, the sun's rays will make their way through and positively influence your hormone function. You can take your 10- or 15-minute breaks outdoors or near a window, or if you're really playing at a high level, you can make a habit of eating your lunch or having your meetings outside.

SUNLIGHT
POWER TIP #3

Only getting sunlight on your skin through the filter of a window might not be the best idea for your health. The sun has a plethora of wavelengths that impact our bodies, but the two you most need to know about are UVA and UVB. UV stands for *ultraviolet,* and these sun rays have long been known to influence our physiology. UVB is the most valuable for human health, as it's the only wavelength that triggers your body to produce vitamin D.

The problem is that UVA has a much longer wavelength than UVB, and it can penetrate through various materials more easily. UVA can move right through the ozone layer, clouds, pollution, and even glass without being filtered out very much. UVB can't make its way through glass very effectively, and it's critical to help balance out the potentially harmful aspects of UVA. It's not that sunlight is inherently bad; it's just the way that we interact with it that can be unhealthy.

We need both UVA *and* UVB, but unhealthy exposure to UVA is what predominantly increases the risk of skin cancer and photoaging of your skin. Getting plenty of natural light through windows during the day is a wonderful thing. Again, that light is being picked up by your optical receptors and sending information to your brain to optimize your circadian timing system. However, exposing yourself to long periods of sunlight directly on your skin through windows should probably be avoided just to be on the safe side.

Also, it's valuable to note that during certain times of the year, depending on where you are in the world, UVB isn't making its way to your body anyway. Generally, during the winter months, it's going to be more challenging to get UVB for most or all of the day. But, again, it depends on where you live. You can find out what time of year and the optimal time of day to get your serving of UVB based on where you are in the world through the bonus Sleep Smarter resources at sleepsmarterbook.com/bonus.

POWER TIP #4

If natural sunlight needs to make its way to your optical receptors for you to get the benefits you've learned about, then sunglasses can be like a 7-foot-tall NBA All-Star and block sunlight's shot at getting to your eyes.

Sunglasses inhibit the natural exposure of light you need to assure healthy hormonal secretions and healthy sleep. It's really as simple as that. As a matter of fact, sunglasses with improper UV protection can be far worse than not wearing sunglasses at all. In bright sunlight, your eyes will naturally try to protect themselves from too much UV light getting in by shrinking the size of the pupils. But when you artificially create darkness over your eyes with standard sunglasses, your pupils open up *wide* and allow in even more potentially harmful UV light.

So try to avoid wearing shades in the sun just for the sake of fashion. If you're going to wear them for temporary eye protection, then make sure that they are truly UV protective by checking with the manufacturer before buying. This can be especially important if you do any snow-based winter sports to help you avoid "sunburn of the eye," also known as *photokeratitis.*

If your future's so bright you have to wear shades, I get it. Just find a healthy way to keep it in balance.

POWER TIP #5

In emergency situations, where you are chained like a prisoner in the cubical dungeon, there are specially designed light boxes, visors, and other gadgets that simulate sunlight. These are often prescribed to treat seasonal affective disorder (SAD), a form of depression that tends to occur during the darker winter months. You can find a list of the best phototherapy devices in the Sleep Smarter bonus resource guide as well. These items are definitely a viable "hack" when you need it, but, remember, you are more powerful than you know to make healthy changes in your life and get yourself the natural sunlight you need. Although these devices are clinically proven to be helpful, even the best light box won't give you as much phototherapy benefit as 30 minutes outside on even an overcast day.

CHAPTER 3

AVOID SCREENS BEFORE BEDTIME

Cutting out some screen time at night is likely the number one thing you can do to improve your sleep *quality* immediately. Computers, iPads, televisions, smartphones, etc., kick out a sleep-sucking blue spectrum of light that can give you major sleep problems. The artificial blue light emitted by electronic screens triggers your body to produce more daytime hormones (such as cortisol) and disorients your body's natural preparation for sleep.

It can be hard to realize just how powerful the artificial blue light is when you're looking into your device in close proximity. Up close, you see a whole world of colors. Yet if the room is dark enough and you take a step back, you can see clearly that the hypnotic blue emanates farther and stronger than any other hue. A good example of this is when you're driving down your neighborhood street at night and you see that majestic blue light beaming out of people's windows. You're probably like a) I wonder what they're watching? or b) I wonder if they're getting abducted by aliens? That blue light is tenacious, and what it's doing to your sleep is really out of this world.

Researchers at Brigham and Women's Hospital in Boston found that the use of light-emitting electronic devices in the hours before bedtime can adversely impact overall health, alertness, and the circadian clock that synchronizes the daily rhythm of sleep. In the study, nighttime iPad readers took longer to fall asleep, felt less sleepy at night, and had shorter REM sleep compared to test subjects who were assigned to read regular printed books. The iPad readers also secreted less melatonin, which, as you know, has a huge impact on sleep quality. What's really vital to note is that they were also more tired than book readers the following day, even if both got a full 8 hours of sleep.

Mariana Figueiro, PhD, of the Lighting Research Center at Rensselaer Polytechnic Institute in Troy, New York, and her team showed that just 2 hours of computer screen time before bed was enough to significantly suppress people's nighttime release of melatonin. When your melatonin secretion is thrown off, it will intrinsically throw off your normal sleep cycle.

Dr. Figueiro also noted that if this nighttime device usage happened on a long-term basis, it could lead to a chronic disruption of circadian rhythms. As a result, the likelihood of serious health issues can skyrocket.

It's important to remember that our cultural use of these electronic devices has been possible for only a few short decades—first with the advent of television, and then really exploding with the invention of laptops, tablets, and smartphones more recently. Millions of years of evolution versus a couple decades of late-night meandering doesn't favor our ability to adapt to this anytime soon.

As human beings, we are literally not designed to stare into the type of light emanating from these devices. When it comes to nighttime usage, we want to be like the little girl in *Poltergeist* and "stay away from the light." (Side note: That movie still creeps me out.)

Of course, we have work to do, and the technology we have available to us today is amazing. We just need to have more awareness and more respect for our body's natural processes so that we can use our devices more wisely.

WHY IS THIS SO HARD?

I recently did a presentation for the corporate employees of one of the largest banks in the United States. The workshop was on boosting employee performance, and, of course, sleeping smarter was a big part of the equation.

Everyone was having an awesome time . . . laughing, learning, and lots of participation. Then it came to the section where we discussed the hazardous effects of hyper-exposure to lights at night, and something interesting happened.

The audience really "got it" when it came to understanding why this mattered so much. But when I asked them what they could do instead of being on their devices before bed, this room full of intelligent adults looked confused and began looking around to see if anyone else knew the answer. It seemed that these people had forgotten what else they could do in life besides using technology before they went to bed.

Then, after a few seconds of bewilderment and silence, one brave woman to my left slowly raised her hand halfway up to give her best shot of answering the question of what we could do besides being on our devices at night before bed. She shyly said, "Read a book?" Notice, it was in the form of a question and not a statement because, again, many of us have forgotten what we can do at night besides being on our tech.

I loudly reaffirmed her unconfident, *Jeopardy*-like answer, saying, "Yes, you can read a book!" That gave another woman on the other side of the room the courage to put her hand up and say, "You can talk to your spouse?" Again, with a question mark behind it, but it was enough for me. I joyously shouted, "Yes, you can talk to your spouse! You can actually talk to a real person, as crazy as it sounds." The audience laughed, and we went on with the presentation. We dove into more strategies to enjoy our lives outside of our devices, but it was a harsh reminder to me that this issue was deeper than just knowing what to do. The bigger issue is that we are actually addicted.

A SPECIAL KIND OF HIGH

When I say we are addicted to technology, this is not just a theory. We really are. And we are hardwired to be that way.

It's not that we are hardwired to the technology itself; it's that we are hardwired to continue to seek.

There's a powerful chemical your body produces called *dopamine*.

Dopamine was once believed to control the "pleasure" systems of the brain. It was thought that dopamine makes you feel enjoyment and pleasure, which therefore motivates you to *seek out* certain behaviors (such as food, sex, and drugs). What scientists have recently discovered is that dopamine is not about pleasure at all. The pleasure is an end result that we receive from the opioid system. Dopamine is a brain chemical that's all about *seeking*. It's about the hunt. It's about finding out what's coming next. And the Internet is a perfect trap for a brain that loves the slow drip of dopamine.

Have you ever gone to Google, or Yahoo, or YouTube and typed in a search for one thing, and then an hour later you have found yourself watching or reading about something totally different?

Have you ever said, "I'll just check my Facebook *for a minute*," or "I'll just check Twitter *for a minute*," or "I'll just check Instagram *for a minute*," and then 30 minutes later you've found yourself sucked into the Internet black hole?

This has happened to practically everyone who's ever been online. The Internet is designed perfectly for the seeking brain and dopamine because there's essentially an infinite amount of data you can "discover" there.

Seeking wouldn't be much without a reward, and the opioid system (basically built-in drugs that make you feel good) follows right behind your Internet search. It's literally like instant gratification. With each new follower you get a notification about, each new "Like" you get from one of your posts, each new photo you scroll past on Instagram, your brain gets a little opioid hit because it discovered something—followed again by more dopamine because it wants to see what's next.

This is a really rudimentary understanding of how your brain responds to your favorite technologies, but hopefully you can see how a vicious circle gets created. This knowledge about dopamine starts to explain how we grown-ups can be as tied to our devices as children with their favorite toys.

WAKE ME UP BEFORE YOU GO-GO

The seeking activity of dopamine isn't the only thing keeping us up. Dopamine itself is tied to being alert and being awake. Drugs that increase levels of dopamine in the brain (including drugs like cocaine, amphetamines, meth, and Ritalin) also increase feelings of wakefulness. A study published by Stanford University found that eliminating the dopamine transporters in mice (which enabled dopamine to stick around longer in their systems) resulted in mice that sleep a lot less.

Dopamine is tied to motivation and alertness, whereas serotonin is tied to contentment and relaxation. These two are operating on two different channels in your body—and which one you're tuned into depends on whether you're watching your television before bed or not.

Balancing your neurotransmitters and hormones is a huge piece to getting amazing sleep at night.

HOW TO TAKE BACK YOUR BRAIN

Many people might remember the commercial from the '80s exemplifying the dangers of doing drugs. The actor shows an egg to the camera and says, "This is your brain." He cracks the egg open and drops it into a hot frying pan. The egg begins to sizzle and he says, "This is your brain on drugs. Any questions?"

That was enough to make me steer clear of drugs, but it was also enough to make me more cautious of eating omelets.

Those anti-drug commercials had a great message and were extremely powerful. But they missed a huge point that we are now aware of today: *Your brain is the greatest drug producer on the planet.* Opioids, serotonin, dopamine, adrenaline, made to order when we knowingly or unknowingly engage in certain lifestyle factors. Most drugs hack into the chemical pathways that your body already has; that's how they're even able to work. Then they artificially stimulate them. This is exactly how your favorite electronic devices work as well.

I'm not in any way saying that you need to be a Luddite and not use your awesome tech devices. I love my smartphone, laptop, etc. These things enable me to reach so many people, to learn faster, and to do it from practically anywhere in the world. It's simply that we need to put these things in a more intelligent place in our lives so that we can continue controlling them, instead of having them control us.

Awareness is the biggest key. Just realizing what's happening in your brain as you're scrolling through Facebook starts to break the old pattern. When you realize what your brain is doing, you basically catch yourself in the act of seeking. When you catch yourself inching close to the edge of the Internet black hole, it's important that you instantly change your behavior because the brain likes to create patterns. And if you continue to do the same thing, it will only make that behavior stronger.

Get up, go get a glass of water, or go and give someone you love a hug. If you have kids, go and love on them, do some stretching (you'll learn about the benefits of bodywork on sleep in Chapter 19), call someone on the phone, or turn on your favorite music. There are so many things you can do to break the addiction. The important thing is that you do something to break the cycle if you have even an inkling that using your devices before sleep could be causing you sleep problems.

There are many other powerhouse tips, insights, and strategies in this book that you can use to your advantage. This chapter covers one of the more challenging keys to sleeping smarter, and although breaking the habit of being on your devices before bed can be a bit more demanding at first, it's definitely one that's worth mastering.

The reality is, we live in a different world today than our parents and grandparents did just a few decades ago, and situations aren't always going to be conducive to being away from our devices late at night. In the *Power Tips* section you're going to get some great hacks that you can use if you're going to be up a little later for an event, family movie night, work, or whatever else might be on the horizon from time to time.

Remember, enjoyment is a huge key to breaking out of the bonds of technology before you go to bed. You can't say, "Okay, tonight I'm going to get off of the computer a couple of hours before I go to bed. Ha-ha! I'm the boss of you, Internet!" and then sit there and twiddle your thumbs. That's a surefire way to get the detox symptoms called the Internet jitters. If you're going to make a new standard to be off of the devices before bed to set you up for a great night's sleep, that time has to be replaced with something you enjoy equally or even more than being on your device. Music, good company, reading, whatever it may be—you have to test and find what fills that space best for you. I'll definitely provide you with some powerful ideas to add to the mix along the way!

◇ ◇ ◇ ◇

SCREEN PROTECTION
POWER TIP #1

If you want to give your body the deep sleep it needs, make it a mandate to turn off all screens at least 90 minutes before bedtime in order to allow melatonin and cortisol levels to normalize. If you ignore this and continue to have problems sleeping, I promise you Jimmy Fallon is not going to pay your hospital bills.

SCREEN PROTECTION
POWER TIP #2

Use an alternative medium for nighttime activity. Remember those papery things called books we talked about? You can actually open one of those ancient relics and enjoy consuming a great story, inspiration, or education that way. And remember when people actually talked to each other face-to-face? You can talk to the people in your life, listen to how their day went, and find out what they're excited about and what they may be struggling with. They can obviously do the same for you, too. In our world, where we're more connected than ever before in some ways, we are often desperately lacking connection in others. Getting off our electronic devices, having a conversation, and showing affection is vital to our long-term health and well-being.

SCREEN PROTECTION
POWER TIP #3

Turn off the cues. Behavioral psychologist Susan Weinschenk, PhD, says, "One of the most important things you can do to prevent or stop a dopamine loop, and be more productive (and get better sleep!), is to turn off the cues. Adjust the settings on your cell phone and on your laptop, desktop, or tablet so that you don't receive the automatic notifications. Automatic notifications are touted as wonderful features of hardware, software, and apps. But they are actually causing you to be like a rat in a cage." If you want to get the best sleep possible, and take back control of your brain, turning off as many visual and auditory cues as you can will be an instant game-changer.

SCREEN PROTECTION
POWER TIP #4

Use a blue light blocker. Extenuating circumstances come up, and you may need to be on your computer later than you want. This is where cool advancements in technology can come in to help smooth things out. On my Mac, I have a free application called f.lux that automatically eliminates the problematic blue light from my computer screen at a certain time each day (you can get similar things for your smartphone and other devices, too—just check out my Sleep Smarter bonus resource guide at sleepsmarterbook.com/bonus for some of the best options). But, again, the best solution is to shut down the technology at least 90 minutes before bed if you're serious about getting great sleep. If that's not feasible, this is a tool you can use that can definitely help you along the way.

You can also find glasses that block blue light in a similar fashion. These are great for other activities outside of being on the computer to help encourage your body to produce more melatonin at night.

If you're really passionate about this stuff, and don't mind looking like someone from the future, then you can rock these glasses that block blue light and give everything a much safer, softer, orange tint. They're similar to the glasses that Brad and Angelina wore in the movie *Mr. and Mrs. Smith* during an epic fight scene. If you get the cheap ones, then you won't look that cool . . . but hey, this is for science, not social points. Just check out the bonus resource guide to see the selection of my favorite sleep-protecting shades as well as many other resources to help you begin sleeping smarter tonight.

CHAPTER 4

HAVE A CAFFEINE CURFEW

Caffeine is a powerful nervous system stimulant. If your nervous system is lit up like a Christmas tree, you can forget about getting high-quality sleep.

The reality is, people like coffee. It is what it is. We just have to learn how to navigate our consumption of coffee and other caffeinated goodies to make sure that we're still getting the best sleep possible.

A study published in the *Journal of Clinical Sleep Medicine* shared some critical insights about the effect of caffeine on sleep that you need to know about. The lead author of the study, Christopher Drake, PhD, associate professor of psychiatry and behavioral neurosciences at Wayne State University School of Medicine in Detroit, says, "Drinking a big cup of coffee on the way home from work can lead to negative effects on sleep, just as if someone were to consume caffeine closer to bedtime."

What the study discovered was that participants given caffeine at different times (immediately before bed, 3 hours before bed, and 6 hours before bed) all showed significant measurable disruptions in their sleep. What this means is that not only is it not a good idea to have caffeine right before bedtime, but having a cup of coffee or caffeinated tea even as much as 6 hours before bed can cause sleep troubles.

What's fascinating about this study is that sleep disturbance was measured in two ways: objectively, by means of a sleep monitor used at home, and subjectively, from diaries kept by the participants. When the participants consumed caffeine 6 hours before bedtime, they had a measurable objective loss of *1 hour* of sleep shown via sleep monitor. The crazy part is that the participants didn't note any subjective difference with their sleep in their sleep journal. Even though they physiologically lost sleep because of the caffeine, they didn't consciously know it at first! To their own knowledge they were fast asleep, though they weren't actually dipping into normal ranges of REM and deep sleep according to the sleep monitor.

This is exactly how the vicious cycle of sleep deprivation gets started. Not getting enough deep sleep due to caffeine consumption inevitably makes us more tired. Being tired makes us want more caffeine. And extra consumption of caffeine will, in turn, make our sleep problems worse. We need to have a strategy to break this vicious cycle to ensure that we're getting the sleep our bodies deserve.

LIVING THE HALF-LIFE

So here's the real deal about caffeine. First of all, the places that caffeine comes from are typically delicious: coffee, chocolate, tea, etc. Not only are they tasty, but caffeine also has a natural affinity with the human body. It can really get our body and mind in a positive place. This is why caffeine can be so addictive.

Caffeine doesn't "give you energy" in the way that most people believe. All day everyday while you're awake, neurons in your brain are firing and producing a neurotransmitter by-product known as *adenosine*. Please understand, adenosine is more than a simple waste product. Your nervous system is constantly monitoring for adenosine in your body, because once the levels of it rise to a certain point in your brain and spinal cord, your body starts to nudge you to go to sleep (or at least to relax). Then, in comes the caffeine . . .

Caffeine has the unique ability to fit into receptor sites in your body for adenosine because it's so structurally similar to the real thing. Normally, when your receptor sites are filled with real adenosine, your body shifts into rest mode. The issue with caffeine going into those receptors is that it simply sits there like a distant relative overextending their stay on your couch. It doesn't actually turn on functions, like adenosine would, to make you tired. As a result, your brain and body are still trucking along and you don't realize that you're actually sleepy. Pretty cool in some ways, but hopefully you can see where this could become a big problem.

Your body is still producing more and more adenosine because of all the "awake" activities you're doing, but the adenosine never gets properly metabolized. As a result, your body literally has to change the way it normally functions, stress hormone levels increase in your system, and your brain and organs get overworked because they aren't getting the accurate cues to rest and recover.

Because of caffeine's long-term effects, it can take several days for its aftermath to wear off. Caffeine has a half-life of around 5 to 8 hours (depending upon your unique biochemical makeup). *Half-life* essentially means that after a specific amount of time (say, 8 hours), half of the substance is still active in your system. So, using the 8-hour half-life as an example, if you consumed 200 milligrams of caffeine (which is equivalent to about one or two cups of standard coffee), after 8 hours, you'd have half of it (or 100 milligrams) active in your system; after another 8 hours, you'd have 50 milligrams; after another 8 hours, it would be 25 milligrams; and so on. This is why having caffeine even 6 hours out from bedtime still caused sleep disturbances in the study.

NICE PARTY TRICK

Caffeine doesn't just affect your nervous system; it affects your endocrine system, too. Caffeine provokes your adrenal glands to produce two anti-sleep hormones: adrenaline and cortisol.

Cortisol we've covered a bit earlier, but adrenaline is something you probably already know about. When we talk about adrenaline, we're talking about fight-or-flight, get-up-and-go, Dwayne "The Rock" Johnson movie, built-in excitement! Guns blazing, tanks, walking away from the explosion in slow motion, the whole 9 yards. Adrenaline is an incredible part of our physiology that allows us to tap into our greatest strengths. Throughout evolution, adrenaline enabled us to either fight off a threat or run for the hills.

Today we are activating that system in a whole new way—through mental and emotional stress (which we'll talk about in Chapter 16) and through the haphazard use of substances like caffeine that intrinsically have side effects.

Though adrenaline can be temporarily entertaining, there's also a big downside. With a spike in stress hormone production there will also come *the crash*. You don't go back to the baseline you were at before the adrenaline spike; you go below it. You tend to feel more tired, have more brain fog, and feel even more irritable than before the adrenaline did its little party trick. While living in the crash, even the nicest person will want to body slam someone unless they are handing them a cup of coffee before talking.

Sue: "Good morning, Jane!"

Jane: "You are not allowed to speak yet. Where's my coffee?"

Jane: (Drinks coffee) "Okay, now you may speak."

Again, caffeine has its perks, but it also has its downside. Because of its effects on our physiology, we can quickly become dependent and not even know it.

CAFFEINE, I WANT TO SEE OTHER PEOPLE . . .

Recently I had the opportunity to work with a really amazing celebrity client. We'll call her Sasha (but her real name was even cooler than that). Sasha is a high-performing, highly successful woman who worked hard to build an empire for herself and her family. She really seemed to have it all, and she knew that she did, but there was one thing that was bothering her in the back of her mind.

Sasha didn't like the idea that something outside of herself had control over her life. She worked on herself and her career for years to really show people what was possible, and that you really can overcome anything. But, no matter how many times she tried to break up with coffee, it just kept finessing its way back into her life.

She loved coffee. She loved the way it made her feel. But she didn't love what would happen to her if she didn't have her coffee. Headaches, low mood, irritation with people she loved dearly. She knew this wasn't normal. She was a big fan of my podcast, *The Model Health Show*, so she thought she'd reach out to me for help.

It was a pleasure working with her because she already knew a lot about health. I was able to provide her with the necessary action steps to get her what she wanted, though what she really needed was straight talk about why she couldn't do this on her own: She was addicted.

She lost track of what it was like to feel like herself and needed coffee to feel "normal." When she tried to break up with coffee in the past, the hallmark symptom she experienced was crushing headaches. Caffeine causes something called *vasoconstriction*—essentially a tightening or narrowing of your blood vessels. If your body is conditioned to having caffeine, and suddenly you stop taking it, you will likely experience a significant shock from something called *vasodilation*—an instant widening of the blood vessels.

Suddenly, where blood flow was once restricted, blood comes rushing in and pushing through more freely. This is typically felt most in the head and neck region and, like migraines, can manifest as a *hemicrania*, or a headache on only one side of the head.

Whatever way you slice it, a caffeine headache can be the pits. And add to that the lower energy and lack of focus, and you have someone fiending for a pot of coffee in a hurry. (Keep in mind, this is in no way a bash against caffeine; I'm actually a fan of caffeine if used intelligently.) In Sasha's case, her addiction had taken over her life. So here's what we did to fix it.

Instead of going cold turkey and just not having her coffee in the morning, we strategized to soften the impact by using caffeine, but from another source and at a lower amount. I had her swap out her coffee for a strong caffeinated tea (like Earl Grey, pu-erh, yerba maté, or English breakfast) that has a nice lick of caffeine, but only one-third to one-half the amount that she would find in coffee. I told her she could even double up on the amount of tea for the first few days, because it's not just about the caffeine itself, it also matters what form it is in. Caffeine from different substances impacts the body differently. The source, processing, and consumption method of any caffeinated product will determine how much caffeine your body receives and how quickly your body will metabolize it.

Next, I had her make sure that she did undergo this process during a period of a few days when she didn't have a lot of work on her plate. She needed to give herself permission to take it easy, de-stress, and relax a bit. Massage is great for this, as is sleeping a little more, taking a relaxing bath, or going for a swim.

Exercise helped as well. I'm not talking about going beast mode in the gym, but just some peaceful walks in nature, a little restorative yoga, and anything else along those lines as long as it wasn't too stressful.

To help flush out metabolic wastes and dilute the coffee residues faster, I had her increase her water intake a bit and add in a little high-quality sea salt because the kidneys are constantly excreting both salt and fluid as they're working to change blood chemistry.

Fiber was another important adjunct combined with the increase in fluid intake. A lot of people lean on coffee for the epic bowel movements it can stimulate. Having a temporary reduction in the gusto of your digestion is normal when you're breaking the coffee habit, but upping your fiber and water intake will help move things along (pun totally intended).

The accountability of having me cheering her on was helpful, too. If you are ever stuck in your life, never underestimate the power of accountability and allowing other people to support and believe in you.

It took about 5 days until she felt fully emancipated from the clutches of her roasted bean romance. She told me that she wasn't feeling like her usual fabulous self for those days, but the process was one-tenth as difficult as it was before, and she knew that it was only temporary.

After the process was over, she said she couldn't be happier. She felt renewed and in control of her mind and body. There really isn't much that's more valuable than that.

Today, she is looking, feeling, and performing better than ever. She and coffee see each other from time to time, but they are no longer in a stressful relationship. Sleep is better, digestion is better, and life is better overall.

It's not that coffee is "bad" in the first place; the issue is what can happen with haphazard use over time. The real challenge is that millions of people aren't just having one serving of caffeine a day; they're having many. We also don't realize when we pick up the habit that our bodies become jaded to the energizing benefits of caffeine. This can happen in as little as

12 days. So, what do we do when we don't notice a strong or consistent enough buzz? We drink more, of course!

The reality is that caffeine is a powerful stimulant, and it can be a wonderfully pleasant part of our lives, if we respect it as such. We need to rewire our bodies to use it on a regular, yet cyclical basis so that we can really get the most bang for the buck.

We know now how caffeine works, and the deleterious effects it can have on our sleep. Now here are some tips to help ensure that caffeine works for—and not against—you.

◇ ◇ ◇ ◇

SMART CAFFEINE
POWER TIP #1

Set an unbreakable caffeine curfew to make sure your body has time to remove the majority of it from your system before bedtime. For most people, that's generally going to be before 2:00 p.m. But, if you're really sensitive to caffeine, you might want to make your curfew even earlier, or possibly avoid caffeine altogether.

SMART CAFFEINE
POWER TIP #2

As you learned in Chapter 2, cortisol plays an important role in managing your body's daily rhythms. Your body's hormonal clock should be producing higher levels of cortisol in the morning and very low levels at night. If you have found that your morning cortisol is lower than normal, or that your hormonal clock is flipped completely upside down overall, a little smart use of caffeine can help to put things back on track.

Since caffeine incites your body's production of cortisol, it can be utilized first thing in the morning to encourage a cortisol boost. If you're a generally healthy individual and not physiologically dependent on caffeine, this could help to set your circadian timing system to produce a little more cortisol during the day and a little less at night. If you have adrenal issues, be sure to check with your physician to make sure that caffeine is safe for you to use.

Products containing caffeine are among the top five most traded commodities in the world because people love them so much. But just because you can get it without a prescription does not mean that it's open season on guzzling hot cocoa and java.

SMART CAFFEINE
POWER TIP #3

Caffeine can even be used strategically to enhance metabolism, increase alertness and focus, and even improve liver function if used in the right way. These are additional reasons why it's important not to throw the baby out with the bathwater and negate the potential benefits of caffeine. As you've learned, your body will down-regulate its response to caffeine over time. To maximize your body's potential benefit from caffeine, it has to be cycled. There are several ways of going about this. I'm going to share three with you:

1. Go 2 days on and 3 days off. If you're a healthy, nonaddicted person using caffeine, it can be cleared from your system nicely after 3 days. When you have it again, you'll notice the same benefits as you did during the initial days you used it.

2. Go 2 months on, 1 month off. This is reasonable if you're using a small to moderate amount of caffeine daily (200 milligrams or less), as in a cup or two of black coffee or tea, or a pre-workout supplement. Using more caffeine than this can lead to withdrawal symptoms for the first few days after discontinued use.

3. Go full on as needed. This is where the magical, "when we first met," experience can happen with coffee and caffeine. On most days, ignore it; live your life normally, without caffeine. But when you need it, go full on into your love affair. Now when I say you "need it," I'm talking about when you have a performance, a big project, or something that is really important (but short in duration, so your indulgence won't be more than a couple of days). Use caffeine as a boost, not a crutch, and you'll be able to truly enjoy its benefits while still sleeping like a champion.

CHAPTER 5

BE COOL

I remember during ridiculously hot summers, my parents wouldn't turn the air conditioner up so that they could "save" on the utility bill. Well, I can tell you that I sweated off a lot of pounds those summers, tossing and turning in my bed upstairs (oh, and heat rises by the way), trying to sleep through the heat. I didn't sleep well then because the temperature of our bodies has a very strong impact on our ability to sleep.

Something called *thermoregulation* heavily influences your body's sleep cycles. Contrary to popular belief, your body temperature doesn't stay uniformly 98.6°F. That is merely an average. Your body temperature cycles from about 1 degree below to 1 degree above this average over the course of the day. When it's time for your body to rest, there is an automatic drop in your core body temperature to help initiate sleep. If the temperature in your environment stays too high, then it can be a bit of a physiological challenge for your body to get into the ideal state for restful sleep.

Studies have found that the optimal room temperature for sleep is really quite cool at around 60° to 68°F. Anything too far above or below this range will likely cause some difficulty sleeping.

To take this discovery even further, studies have shown that insomniacs (individuals with chronic sleep issues) tend to have a significantly warmer

NORMAL HUMAN BODY TEMPERATURES
THROUGHOUT THE DAY

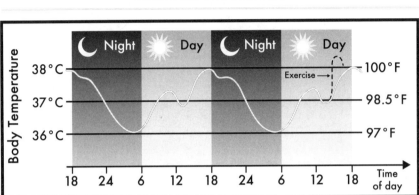

body temperature than normal right before bed. To help combat this issue, researchers at the University of Pittsburgh School of Medicine conducted a study to find a way to cool insomniacs off and then determine if that did, indeed, have an impact on their overall sleep quality.

During the study the test subjects were fitted with "cooling caps" that contained circulating water at cool temperatures. What the researchers discovered by the end of the study was pretty shocking. When the participants wore the cooling caps, they fell asleep *even faster* than people without sleep disorders. With the caps, the insomniacs took about 13 minutes to fall asleep, compared to 16 minutes for the healthy control group. What's also interesting is that the patients diagnosed with insomnia ended up sleeping for 89 percent of the time they were in bed, which was the exact amount of time the healthy control group slept in bed.

This study demonstrated that cooling the body temperature helped to "balance out" those with chronic sleep struggles with a 75 percent success rate. There are very few treatments on the market that even come close to this in effectiveness, but by utilizing the tips at the end of the chapter, we can all gain a lot of benefit from it.

YOUR INTERNAL THERMOSTAT

Being warmer than normal at night will inherently lead to a heightened state of arousal and a struggle to fall asleep while your body tries to reset its internal thermostat.

So where is this internal thermostat anyway? Can it actually be changed to a different setting?

To find your body's internal thermostat, you have to go back to our understanding of the master gland, the hypothalamus. The hypothalamus actually integrates the functions of your nervous system (which senses the internal and external temperature) and your endocrine system (which secretes specific hormones to either induce sleep or keep you awake). Your hypothalamus is like the coach of your cellular basketball team.

If your "coach" is treated well—given a nice salary of nutrition, plenty of healthy movement, and not overstressed—chances are it can keep everyone in line, achieving the greatest results possible. Think the "Zen Master," Phil Jackson. He managed stress like a pro and brought the best out of his "body" of players.

On the other hand, if the coach is unhealthy, underpaid, overworked, and lacking proper support, it can start miscommunicating the roles of the team, and then the whole thing can fall apart fast. This is why the health and support of your brain is so important.

Your hypothalamus is part of a very significant system in your body known as the *hypothalamic-pituitary-adrenal axis*, or HPA axis for short. The HPA axis is critical in normal hormone function, sexual function, managing body weight, and more. The most important takeaway here is that the HPA axis is your body's number one system for managing stress.

The previously mentioned study on insomniacs also found that the test subjects experienced greater levels of anticipatory anxiety than normal test subjects. Their *worry* and *stress* over sleeping were higher, which likely contributed to their increase in core body temperature. It's not just the environment that needs to be cool; you need to be cool, too (as in your mental and emotional state). Your HPA axis deals with the overall stress load in your life. From work, to relationships, to nutrition, to your exercise, your HPA axis manages it all.

As a result of your body's efforts to battle perceived threats, stress can arouse your system, elevate your body temperature, and unwittingly disrupt your sleep. You absolutely must have a strategy to manage stress in our high-stress world today, or you can sleep in an igloo and still not be cool enough. We'll talk about some life-changing stress-management tools coming up in Chapter 16. For now, let's get the environment around you optimized for the best sleep possible, so that you have a smart, well-rounded approach to the free throw line. Swish!

◇ ◇ ◇ ◇

POWER TIP #1

Make sure that the temperature in your bedroom stays close to the recommended 68°F at night. For some people, this is just right, but others may have images of Jack Frost and Frosty the Snowman. Trust me (and the science), you will sleep better if you're a little cooler; just don't overdo it—60°F is the recommended minimum. You can still have your covers and pj's, but don't overdo that either or you'll keep your body temperature too high (chances are your lover or would-be lover doesn't want to sleep next to a flannel-clad, multiple-layered lumberjack at night anyway). Get a nice, cool environment in your room and snuggle up to sleep more soundly.

POWER TIP #2

If you have trouble falling asleep, try taking a warm bath 1½ to 2 hours before hitting the sack. This may seem counterintuitive, but while your core temperature will increase from the bath, it will fall accordingly and level out a little cooler right around the time you turn in for the night. Many parents know that this is the secret method for helping young kids fall asleep and *stay* asleep at night.

POWER TIP #3

There are mattress pads you can use that may help regulate your body temperature. These specially designed pads can fit securely over one or both sides of your existing mattress. My friend and *New York Times* bestselling author Kelly Starrett, DPT, swears by his mattress pad to keep him a little cooler than his wife at night. He said it was a game changer for him. You can check out the cooling pads we recommend in the Sleep Smarter bonus resource guide at sleepsmarterbook.com/bonus.

Eus van Someren, PhD, and colleagues at the Netherlands Institute for Neuroscience in Amsterdam found that though sleeping in a cooler environment is valuable overall, every person should be "perfectly comfortable." This level of perfect comfort is going to be unique to you. Cooling the room off is a must, but some people will feel great all night with a fluffy comforter, some with just a few bed sheets, and some would feel even better using an additional cooling pad like Dr. Starrett does.

KEEP IT COOL
POWER TIP #4

Rock socks. Even though the room temperature will ideally be cooler to induce great sleep, this can trigger sleeplessness in some people because their extremities are too cold. This is because blood flow is the primary method of distributing heat throughout the body. If your hands and feet are too cold, it could be a sign of poor circulation. The solution: Wear a pair of warm socks to bed if you need to. Some people are naturally more warm-bodied and prefer to be barefoot, so test it out and see what works best for you.

CHAPTER 6

GET TO BED AT
THE RIGHT TIME

You can literally get amplified benefits of sleep by sleeping at the right hours. Renowned neurologist Kulreet Chaudhary, MD, says, "Timing your sleep is like timing an investment in the stock market—it doesn't matter how much you invest, it matters *when* you invest."

It's been shown that human beings get the most beneficial hormonal secretions and recovery by sleeping during the hours of 10:00 p.m. to 2:00 a.m. This is what I call *money time*.

You get the most rejuvenating effects during this period, and any sleep that you get in addition is a nice bonus. This is based on the seemingly lost realization that we humans are a part of nature, and when the lights go out on the planet, that's a cue from the universe that it's time for us to turn down, too.

Today, however, we can trump nature and light up our house like a Las Vegas stripper sign. We can be up until 2:00 a.m. doing the laptop lap dance and not even think twice about it.

Because of our typical living conditions today, it can be hard for us to realize that this is abnormal.

We are literally designed to go to sleep within a few hours after it gets dark, so if you've made a habit of ignoring this innate law, it's time to take action to readjust.

In our discussion on sunlight exposure in Chapter 2, we found that our body's natural production of hormones is critical to getting the best sleep possible. When you line your sleep up with your natural hormone secretions, the benefits you get from sleep will be exponentially better.

For example, you may be sleeping from 1:00 a.m. to 9:00 a.m. and getting 8 hours of sleep, but you are missing out on most of that money time when the beneficial hormone secretions are at their highest. Melatonin, human growth hormone (HGH), and more are secreted in their strongest doses when your sleep is lined up properly. Want to stay young and vibrant longer? Then you need to know that you get the best dose of HGH, the "youth hormone," if you're sleeping during those prime-time hours.

Some people get 8 or more hours of sleep but still don't feel well rested when they wake up. Dr. Chaudhary states, "If your body is chronically deprived of the regenerative sleep between 10:00 p.m. and 2:00 a.m., then you may still feel fatigued when you wake up in the morning." Again, this affirms the understanding that it's all about hormone production, and missing out on that money time is not a very smart investment.

THE SECOND WIND

Around 10:00 p.m., your body goes through a transformation following the natural rise in melatonin. The purpose of this transformation is to increase *internal* metabolic energy to repair, strengthen, and rejuvenate your body. Heightened production of antioxidant hormones happens at this time to help protect your DNA from damage, improve your brain function, and more. If you're asleep as normal during this phase, all is well. However, if you're up when 10:00 p.m. rolls around, that increase in metabolic energy can be experienced as a "second wind."

Have you ever had this happen before? After work, around 6:00 or 7:00 p.m., you're tired. You can't wait to hit the sack and get a great night's sleep.

Then 10 o'clock rolls around and you feel wide-awake and ready to do stuff! It's very likely that you have just experienced the energy second wind. It's really not that much different from exercise. People who've done any type of endurance training know that if you keep at it for a certain amount of time, even though you're tired, your body will kick into a second wind and you'll feel energized again and ready to keep going.

Instead of the increased energy being used for necessary internal house-keeping, it was used for you to scroll through Facebook and watch three more episodes of your favorite show on Netflix.

It's important to understand that your body's ability to repair itself, remove free radicals, and maximize hormonal output is greatly inhibited when you allow yourself to stay up and move into that second wind. People who stay up past 10:00 or 11:00 p.m. and dig into that second wind energy often find that they have a harder time falling asleep when they want to. The result can be that you're more fatigued and groggy when you wake up in the morning. But this is only a small slice of what habitually staying up late can do.

THE GRAVEYARD SHIFT

If you stretch this out and live a lifestyle where you're consistently disrupting your body's natural hormone clock, then big problems could be on the horizon. The International Agency for Research on Cancer has now classified overnight shift work as a Group 2A carcinogen. This means that staying up late repeatedly, and working overnight, is a strong enough cancer-causing agent to be lumped in with lead exposure and UVA radiation. That might sound crazy, but there's now a ton of scientific data showing exactly how this happens.

As we have discussed, the antioxidant hormone melatonin has a huge impact on your sleep quality, and it is paramount to your health overall. What's also fascinating about melatonin is that it may be one of the most powerful anti-cancer hormones your body can produce.

Not only is it getting props for being an excellent free radical scavenger, helping to protect your cells and tissues from damage, but it has also been found to protect your body from cancer in another unique way.

The journal of the Federation of American Societies for Experimental Biology (*The FASEB Journal*) published extensive research showing that melatonin has very strong *antiestrogenic* effects. Many breast cancer drugs actually utilize synthetic antiestrogens because of their ability to inhibit breast cancer cell proliferation. Your body is producing one of the strongest antiestrogens every night—*if* you're getting the sleep you really require.

Breast cancer is known to be strongly linked to excessive estrogen activity in the body. Because both men and women produce estrogen, too much estrogen activity, or the abnormal function of estrogen, could trigger significant health challenges. In women it could show up as breast cancer, uterine cancer, and fibroid tumors. In men it could show up as a depression of secondary sex characteristics (things like stunted growth, lack of body hair, or having a lighter voice), an increase in growth of breast tissue (gynecomastia), and cancer as well.

A study published in the *International Journal of Cancer* found that women who worked the overnight shift had a 30 percent greater incidence of breast cancer. Other studies on female nurses who worked overnight found that the greater the number of years they worked the late shift, the more their rates of cancer would skyrocket.

Cancer isn't the only issue that was found to be strongly linked to shift work. Another study reported in the journal *Occupational and Environmental Medicine* found that night shift workers have significantly higher rates of diabetes—especially male workers. Authors of numerous studies suggest that the higher rates of diabetes in shift workers are because of the damaging effects this type of work has on insulin. As mentioned earlier, just one night of sleep deprivation can make you as insulin resistant as a person with type 2 diabetes, but extend that out to when you're not sleeping during the night at all, and you and diabetes will do more than just flirt with each other.

These are just some of the chronic diseases resulting from overnight work that should be a real eye-opener for you. But what about the more obvious things like accidents and injuries from being up late at night?

Well, according to University of British Columbia researchers, working the night shift could nearly double your risk of suffering a workplace injury.

Their study examined data from more than 30,000 people who worked different shifts over the course of 10 years. Due to improvements in job safety, the rate of injury overall went down for people working daytime shifts, but they did not go down for those who were working overnight.

More injuries, more accidents, and a higher rate of mortality are seen consistently for those who are working overnight. So, whether you're staying up late for the purpose of work or the purpose of entertainment, doing this consistently could lead to the graveyard shift showing you exactly what the name really means.

WE HAVE TO FIND ANOTHER WAY

I am very passionate about this particular subject of shift work because some of the most important people in our lives are impacted by it. Our doctors, nurses, law enforcement officers, firefighters, and many others are working these shifts to help keep us safe and our countries in good working order.

The jobs they do are vital. But they're coming at a huge cost. We've already talked about the impact on nurses with the increased rate of breast cancer, but also there is an increased rate of colorectal cancer, obesity, and cardiovascular disease as well. This holds true for doctors, too—the average life span of physicians is up to 10 years less than the general public in some regions.

Research published in the journal *Workplace Health & Safety* found that police officers who work during the night are 14 times more likely to be chronically sleep deprived. And this sleep deprivation was linked with an increased risk of metabolic syndrome—a condition with a variety of symptoms ranging from excess body fat, to high triglycerides (blood fats), to elevated blood pressure and blood sugar levels. Similar health risks are seen in studies with firefighters and many other positions that have overnight work as well.

These are the people entrusted with our health, and our society has been set up in such a way that we are not returning the favor for them. Education about the importance of sleep is a start, but having a proactive strategy to help our shift-working heroes could be the key to seeing less disease and far more years of great health for them.

CAN WE REALLY MAKE UP OUR SLEEP ON THE WEEKENDS?

Now, logically, do you really think you can make up on sleep? There's this interesting term called *sleep debt* that refers to the cumulative effect of not getting enough sleep. The key word here is *cumulative*. The side effects start aggregating and piling up on each other pretty quickly. A short sleep debt, say maybe one night of poor sleep, can be cleaned up by your body rather nicely with good sleep, good nutrition, and smart exercise to help move things along.

However, even a couple nights of poor sleep can have the hormonal Goodfellas knocking at your door to pay back a sleep debt that you simply can't repay. If you keep haphazardly building up the sleep debt, you just might find yourself swimming with the fishes!

Joyce Walsleben, PhD, adjunct associate professor in the department of medicine at New York University's Sleep Disorders Center, points out that making up for lost sleep on the weekend is really too late. She notes, "You've already been irritable and possibly experienced poor reaction times that may have caused accidents. Snoozing late on the weekend can also disrupt your sleep rhythm and make it difficult to go to bed Sunday night, so you'll be starting the next week already in the hole."

She's bringing up the fact that it's really advantageous to have a consistent sleep schedule no matter what day it is. And unless you have a DeLorean, you can't go back in time and undo the mistakes you made when you were trying to live your life sleep deprived.

Think about what you're gaining with more money time sleep rather than what you might be missing out on. Much of what we are doing late at night can be done during the day with some smart planning and prioritization. We all have the same 24 hours—it's really what you do with it that makes all the difference.

Not only do you get added health benefits from getting more money time sleep, but you are also protecting yourself from a whole host of issues that can have you clocking out long before your time. Now, let's get into some specific tips to get that money time sleep your body really deserves.

◇ ◇ ◇ ◇

MONEY TIME
POWER TIP #1

The 10:00 p.m. recommended bed time isn't exact with all of the variation in time zones, daylight saving time, how far you are from the equator, the time of year, etc. If we get too neurotic about the exact time to go to sleep, it can get a little ridiculous. To get the highest-quality sleep possible, you want to aim for getting to bed within a few hours of it getting dark outside.

For most people, this is going to mean somewhere between 9:00 p.m. and 11:00 p.m. most of the year. By doing this, you are giving yourself a huge hormonal advantage. During the winter season, humans would naturally be sleeping more and going to bed a bit earlier. Conversely, during the summer months when the days are longer, you have a bit of a permission slip to stay up later and enjoy the weather a little more. Nature is giving us direct cues on when to sleep; we just need to learn to pay attention to them.

MONEY TIME
POWER TIP #2

To help reset your sleep cycle so that you're actually tired when the optimal bedtime rolls around, make a habit of getting some sunlight as soon as possible when you wake up. This is going to help boost your natural cortisol levels and fully wake your system up. Your body knows what to do, and it will find its natural sleep cycle when you practice good sleep hygiene and follow the tips in this book.

MONEY TIME
POWER TIP #3

If health is your number one priority, then don't work the night shift. If service is your number one priority, and shift work happens to be a part of that, do everything you can to stack the conditions in your favor by following the rest of the Sleep Smarter strategies. Lots of people who would rather not be working overnight tell themselves that it's something they have to do, that they don't have another choice. The reality is you *always* have a choice. As soon as you say something is impossible, that's when you close the door to the hundreds of other opportunities that are a lot closer than you think.

If you had to get a different job and work normal hours to save the life of someone you love, you'd find a way. You'd always find a way. It's just that we tend to settle and get comfortable in our story unless our backs are against the wall and the pain is bad enough. It's a sad reality that most people (but not you!) still continue to forfeit their health and happiness even when the pain *is* bad enough. It's because they've lost connection with what's most important, which is the fact that we are all the most creative, industrious, resourceful beings on the planet when we want to be. The power lies in our decisions, not our circumstances. Once we realize this, the whole game changes for good. Decide to work at normal hours for your health and happiness, and take action in that direction until you make it happen.

MONEY TIME
POWER TIP #4

This tip may be helpful for those who manage shifts and people in major organizations out there. One of the strategies for our overnight workers, like doctors and firefighters, might be to have a specific intense period of overnight work and then a much longer period of having normal sleeping hours. A common practice is for them to work 2 to 3 days a week overnight and then back to normal. The research in the nurses' study found that varying sleep cycles so much during the week was just as harmful over the long term as working overnight for years at a time.

A better approach could be to have 2 months *off* the normal sleep cycle where they're working overnight, and 10 months *on* the natural sleep schedule where their bodies get to be in sync with their natural circadian clocks. Though this is still not ideal, our bodies are incredibly resilient when we're doing things right. This different format, plus following the other tips in this book, could be the key to improving the health of the people who take care of ours.

POWER TIP #5

During normal sleep at night, your body follows a predictable pattern, moving back and forth between deep, restorative sleep (deep sleep) and more alert stages (non-REM) and dreaming (REM sleep). These stages of REM and non-REM sleep come together to form a complete sleep cycle.

Sleep cycles typically last for 90 minutes each and repeat four to six times per night. So, six normal 90-minute sleep cycles would equal 9 total hours of sleep.

Even if you get a full night's sleep, you can still wake up feeling groggy if your alarm goes off during the middle of one of your sleep cycles. To make your mornings better and more energetic, start setting your alarm so that it goes off in accordance with these sleep cycles instead of the standard "8 hours of sleep." For example, if you go to sleep at 10:00 p.m., set your alarm for 5:30 a.m. (for a total of $7^1/_2$ hours of sleep), and you'll likely find that you feel more refreshed when you wake up than if you set the alarm for 6:00 a.m. and interrupted another sleep cycle.

HUMAN SLEEP CYCLES

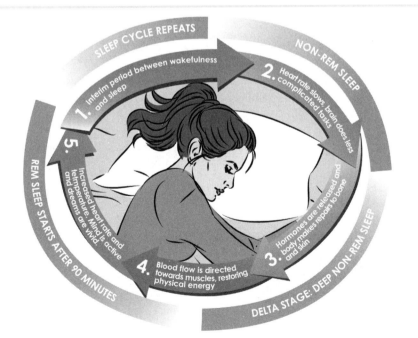

SLEEP CYCLE REPEATS

NON-REM SLEEP

1. Interim period between wakefulness and sleep

2. Heart rate slows, brain does less complicated tasks

3. Hormones are released and body makes repairs to bone and skin

4. Blood flow is directed towards muscles, restoring physical energy

5. Increased heart rate and temperature. Mind is active and dreams are vivid

REM SLEEP STARTS AFTER 90 MINUTES

DELTA STAGE: DEEP NON-REM SLEEP

Alternatively, you can go for an additional sleep cycle if that's what makes you feel best. Again, going to bed at 10:00 p.m. for example, set your alarm for 7:00 a.m. to get that sixth full sleep cycle under your belt. And, here's a great tip if you ever do find yourself in a pinch and need to sleep less than normal. Shoot for getting that minimum of four sleep cycles in for a total of 6 hours. If you have to stay up until 1:00 a.m. (again, not ideal, but it happens), set your alarm for 7:00 a.m., not 7:30 or 8:00 a.m., and you'll likely find that you feel better when you wake up to start your day. Use these sleep hacks for the forces of good, and your body will pay you big dividends in return.

CHAPTER 7

FIX YOUR GUT TO FIX YOUR SLEEP

The food that you eat can dramatically impact the quality of sleep that you get.

Remember, food isn't just food—it's *information*. And the types of food that you eat, along with the nutrients they contain (or lack thereof), automatically incite processes that determine what your body, health, and sleep will look like.

Not only that, the environment in your belly itself can either make or break getting a good night's sleep, so what you're about to learn can really be a game changer for you.

As you discovered in Chapter 2, upwards of 95 percent of your body's serotonin is located in your gut. Serotonin is produced in the *enterochromaffin cells* in the intestinal mucosa. Once it's released, it activates your system to increase intestinal motility. Serotonin literally helps the ebb and flow of your digestion overall.

The obvious sleep connection is that serotonin is the building block for the "get-good-sleep" hormone, melatonin. The not-so-obvious connection is that serotonin, and the health of your digestion, can impact your brain and sleep more powerfully than almost anything you can think of.

Recently, scientists have uncovered that the human gut is a mass of neural tissue, filled with 30 types of neurotransmitters (just like the brain), and found that it does a whole lot more than just help the sandwich you ate make it out to the other side.

Because of the massive amount of brainlike tissue found in the gut, it has rightfully earned the title of being "the second brain." Technically known as the *enteric nervous system*, this second brain consists of around 100 million neurons, more than in either the spinal cord or even the peripheral nervous system. Basically, your belly has the smarts to easily do calculus, but instead it's focused on doing so much more.

To top it all off (and this is the real kicker), the gut has been found to contain at least 400 times more melatonin than the pineal gland in your brain. Research shows that even after a surgical removal of the pineal gland, those levels of melatonin found in the gut remain relatively the same, highlighting how tissues in the gut (in particular the enteroendocrine cells) are extremely effective at producing melatonin themselves. This bona fide sleep hormone can be found in optimal supply in your belly if things are going well. That said, I hope you can start to see that the health of your gut (and everything that happens in there) will always have a tremendous impact on the quality of your sleep.

The vagus nerve has a huge role in bringing this all together. The vagus nerve interfaces with the heart, lungs, and other organs on a pathway straight to your brain. What researchers at UCLA were shocked to find was that about 90 percent of the fibers in the vagus nerve carry information from the gut to the brain and not the other way around. The environment in your gut and the health of your gut is a primary system calling the shots with your brain function. This highlights the fact that what happens in vagus really does not stay in vagus.

YOUR BELLY IS DRIVING YOUR BRAIN
(BUT WHO IS DRIVING YOUR BELLY?)

Researchers at UCLA also discovered that the trillions of bacteria in your gut are continuously communicating with your enteric nervous system (aka your second brain), and researchers from the California Institute of Technology (Caltech) reported that certain bacteria in the gut play an important role in the production of the serotonin that you've been learning about.

You have approximately 10 times more bacteria that live in and on your body than you have human cells, and most of them are camping out in your gut. Now, don't be freaked out. This is exactly how it's supposed to be. We have evolved to have a symbiotic relationship with these bacteria. When in natural balance, they help to regulate your immune system, your digestive system, and even your sleep, as you will find out.

There are bacteria referred to as *friendly flora* that have tremendous resonance with our health. Then there are *unfriendly flora*, or opportunistic bacteria that can cause a lot of damage if things get out of sorts. Yet, even the unfriendly bacteria have a role. Think of the Incredible Hulk in the movie *The Avengers*. He wasn't exactly a nice guy, though he helped the team to win. But if the world was filled with Incredible Hulks, then things would probably go to hell in a handbasket pretty quickly.

It's really the ratio of friendly bacteria to unfriendly bacteria that matters. You want the good guys controlling your ship, because if the bad guys take over, they will keep steering you right to the fast-food drive-thru and causing a ruckus that keeps you up at night.

A study on what happens to your intestinal flora due to irregular sleep patterns was published in the journal *Cell*. Researchers discovered that your circadian timing system influences your bacteria balance. Common experiences like jet lag were enough to create bacterial dysbiosis in the gut, which, in turn, leads to metabolic disorders.

In the study, researchers analyzed fecal samples from people before, during, and after bouts of jet lag from a 10-hour flight spanning multiple time zones. They found that the jet-lagged participants showed an increase in a type of bacteria known to be more prevalent in people with obesity and diabetes. Then the levels of these microbes dropped back to normal once the travelers got back on a regular sleep cycle.

It has been found that your gut bacteria also have a circadian timing system, and there's a virtual "changing of the guard" that happens every night to help keep the good guys in control of your vessel. If you don't sleep, or don't sleep well, then it gives the opportunistic bacteria a chance to take over your gut (and thus, your brain).

Sleep deprivation has been proven (as you'll learn more about in Chapter 13) to lead to poorer food choices and overeating, which both serve to keep the unfriendly bacteria in control. They've got to eat, too!

CHANGE YOUR FOOD, CHANGE YOUR SLEEP

What we've been referring to with this conversation about good and bad bacteria can be described as your *gut microbiome*. To aid in normal serotonin production, melatonin secretion, and optimal hormone function overall, you have to make sure that you avoid things that can damage your microbiome and lead to a hostile takeover.

Some of the things clinically proven to damage or disorient your gut microbiome are:

- **Agricultural chemicals** (pesticides, fungicides, rodenticides): The suffix *cide* means "to kill" by the way!
- **Processed foods:** The excessive sugars are shown to feed pathogenic bacteria.
- **Haphazard or repeated antibiotic use:** Most antibiotics don't care which jersey your bacteria are wearing, they are taking out everybody!
- **Chemical food additives and preservatives:** A lot of times these have no business being in your food.
- **Chlorinated water:** Chlorine is a known antibiotic. Though it's an excellent cleaner, even in small amounts it can damage your bacteria cascade; it's best to get yourself a water filter that removes chlorine if your municipality uses it. You can check out more on getting yourself the ideal water and all the incredible benefits it will have on your body at themodelhealthshow.com/water.

These are several of the main concerns that can lead to gut dysbiosis, but there are other issues as well. Many of the things we've accepted as normal in our society are anything but. We have to take our blinders off and see that the consumption of man-made, processed foods is doing a number on our brain-body connection and damaging our health overall.

For example, on a popular episode of my podcast, *New York Times* bestselling author Sara Gottfried, MD, shared her insights on how things like diet soda can wreak havoc on your gut microbiome. Soda is highly processed and bad enough for you as it is, but she said, "Diet soda may be even worse for you than regular soda—in terms of what it does to your microbiome and metabolism. It can *break* your metabolism." Many people are realizing that just because something has the word "diet" slapped on it doesn't mean that it's good for you. We still have a long way to go in making real, sustainable health information the norm, but no longer falling for marketing catchwords is a huge victory in this mission.

As you can see, it's not just about putting in the good stuff for your sleep and health; it's avoiding the not-so-good stuff that can help ensure that the right things will actually work. So, now let's look at some of the important foods and nutrients that your body (and bacteria) will love to help you get the best sleep possible.

EAT MORE GOOD-SLEEP NUTRIENTS

When it comes to getting the nutrients you need to keep your body and sleep healthy, remember this: Food first. Of course, there are occasions to strategically add in some smart supplementation (as we'll talk about in-depth in Chapter 17 and something special at the end of this chapter as well) to help fill in the nutritional gaps and get things back in line from what can sometimes be a lifetime of deficiency.

The reason food is so paramount to getting these nutrients is that your body has evolved to "recognize" the nutrients that it can extract from whole foods. There's no guarantee that your body is going to readily assimilate the vitamin C from a supplement just because the pill bottle says it's in there. Your cells (and those bacteria in your gut that we've been talking about) are more likely to play nicely with real food that it has evolved eating in one form or another since the beginning of time, than the fancy supplement that was made by Cousin Vinny at the lab last week.

Here are some important good-sleep nutrients you need to ensure you're getting on a regular basis and the best foods to find them in:

Selenium: A deficiency in selenium could play a role in sleep abnormalities.

It's also critical for your immune system function and thyroid function. With selenium, a little bit can go a long way. Great sources are Brazil nuts, sunflower seeds, beef, oysters, chicken, and cremini mushrooms.

Vitamin C: A study published by the Public Library of Science (PLOS) revealed that people with low blood levels of vitamin C had more sleep issues and were more prone to waking up during the night. Excellent sources of vitamin C are superfoods like camu camu berry, amla berry, and acerola cherry, as well as more everyday foods like bell peppers, green leafy vegetables, kiwifruit, strawberries, citrus fruits, and papaya.

Tryptophan: This is a critical nutrient because it's the precursor to your body's serotonin production. Tryptophan is found in turkey, chicken, eggs, sweet potatoes, chia seeds, hemp seeds, bananas, pumpkin seeds, almonds, yogurt, and leafy greens.

Potassium: A study published in the journal *Sleep* found that potassium may be helpful for those who have trouble staying asleep. Bananas are often touted as the best source of potassium, but there are far better sources (especially if you want to avoid the excess sugar). Leafy greens, potatoes, dulse (a mineral-rich sea veggie), broccoli, cremini mushrooms, and avocados are excellent sources of potassium. If you love guacamole, this is probably the best news ever.

Calcium: The journal *European Neurology* published a study showing that disturbances in REM sleep were linked to a calcium deficiency. Great sources of bioavailable calcium are kale, collard greens, mustard greens, sardines, sea veggies, and sesame seeds.

Vitamin D: According to the *Journal of Clinical Sleep Medicine*, there is a strong correlation between vitamin D deficiency and excessive daytime sleepiness. There are a few food sources of vitamin D, such as swordfish, salmon, tuna, mackerel, shiitake mushrooms, and oysters, but the optimal way to get your vitamin D levels up, as the research indicates, is through smart exposure to natural sunlight.

We talked about this thoroughly in Chapter 2, which you can always refer back to if needed. But as you know, it isn't always possible to get the adequate sunlight we need because of where we live and the time of year. This would be a smart place to supplement, at least part of the year, with an intelligently produced vitamin D_3 supplement.

D_3 is the specific type of vitamin D you need. You can check out my favorite sources for vitamin D_3 supplements through the bonus resources guide found at sleepsmarterbook.com/bonus.

Omega-3s: A study conducted by the University of Oxford found that omega-3s can help you get deeper, more restful sleep. Some food sources of omega-3s are chia seeds, pumpkin seeds, hemp seeds, walnuts, halibut, salmon, and flax seeds. A note about omega-3 fatty acids is that they are known to be heat-sensitive, so excessive heat could damage the sensitive oils you are trying to get. This is why opting for cold-processed oils like flax oil, fish oil, and krill oil from a reputable brand is a good idea.

Melatonin: Some foods actually have small amounts of melatonin in them. And some foods have been found to help raise your body's *production* of melatonin. Tart cherries are far and away the food source with the highest amount of melatonin, but there is also a tiny amount found in walnuts, ginger root, and asparagus. Some of the foods that have been found to naturally boost your body's melatonin levels are pineapples (the leader in one particular study), tomatoes, bananas, and oranges.

Vitamin B_6: This essential vitamin helps to modulate your body's stress response and relax your nervous system. Some of the best sources of vitamin B_6 are bananas, yogurt (sugar free and organic, please!), cashews, peanut butter, almonds, avocados, fish, tomatoes, spinach, sweet potatoes, sea veggies, and eggs.

Probiotics and prebiotics: Probiotic supplements are becoming very popular today, but there are also many foods that provide the beneficial flora that can help support healthy digestion. Most long-lived cultures in human history have some form of fermented food or beverage. Here are a few that have stood the test of time: sauerkraut, kimchi, pickles (you can pickle pretty much anything!), miso, yogurt (dairy and nondairy), kefir (dairy and nondairy), and kombucha.

This doesn't mean you should start gobbling down commercial yogurt products, or popping probiotic pills for that matter. The bacteria strains found in these different items vary greatly, and what you may need to heal your gut and heal your digestion may be radically different from what the next person needs. If you suspect that you may have an issue with gut dysbiosis, I highly recommend that you check out the resources at sleepsmarterbook.com/bonus for more targeted information.

Another useful factor in helping the friendly flora to thrive in your system, rather than the unfriendly flora, is the addition of smart *prebiotic* foods. Prebiotics are essentially compounds that aid the growth or activity of probiotics within your system. Proven prebiotic foods for a healthy belly and body are things like Jerusalem artichokes, raw garlic, raw and cooked onions, dandelion greens, and asparagus, just to name a few.

There are many other foods and nutrients that are important for human health. The great thing about eating real foods is that you'll get a whole host of other nutrients that come along with the ones above, all in a delicious, bioavailable form.

It should go without saying that these foods would ideally be organic and minimally processed (especially after learning what chemical additives can do to your gut health). All of these nutrients are incredibly valuable, but there is one more that just might be in a league of its own.

ONE MIGHTY MINERAL

Magnesium is a certified anti-stress mineral. It helps to balance blood sugar, optimize circulation and blood pressure, relax tense muscles, reduce pain, and calm the nervous system. Yet, because it has so many functions, it tends to get depleted from our bodies rather fast.

Magnesium deficiency is likely the number one mineral deficiency in our world today. Estimates show that upwards of 80 percent of the population in the United States is deficient in magnesium. And some experts say that these numbers are actually conservative. Chances are, you're not getting enough magnesium into your system, and getting your magnesium levels up can almost instantly reduce your body's stress load and improve the quality of your sleep.

Not only is magnesium important for optimizing your sleep, it's critical to your health and longevity overall. A study published in the *Journal of Intensive Care Medicine* showed that people deficient in magnesium were twice as likely to die prematurely. I don't know about you, but I don't want to clock out before my time. Optimizing your magnesium levels can be key to living a long, healthy life.

When discussing magnesium, Mark Hyman, MD, director of the Cleveland Clinic Center for Functional Medicine, states, "This critical mineral is actually responsible for over 300 enzyme reactions and is found in all of your tissues—but mainly in your bones, muscles, and brain. You must have it for your cells to make energy, for many different chemical pumps to work, to stabilize membranes, and to help muscles relax."

Magnesium levels can be a serious problem or a serious benefit depending on where you are on the spectrum. This is definitely not something to take lightly.

In addition to the proven impact magnesium has on your body, research shows that one of the central symptoms of magnesium deficiency is chronic insomnia. This is valuable information to know because simply getting your magnesium levels up can have a huge impact on your sleep quality very quickly.

GET IT UP THE SMART WAY

Because of our high-stress world and the way that magnesium is used up in the body, food alone will likely not solve the issue of magnesium deficiency. Supplementation may not be the best method to get your magnesium levels up either. Research has shown that a large percentage of magnesium is lost in the digestive process. So, what do we typically do to compensate with a supplement? Take more, of course!

The problem is that taking too much of a low-budget internal magnesium supplement can have you sprinting to the bathroom faster than Usain Bolt. Magnesium actually pulls more water to your bowels, which can lead to one or many unexpected bathroom breaks. In layman's terms: You might end up with disaster pants.

Quality is everything when it comes to your magnesium sources. High-quality supplementation can be helpful in small amounts, as well as a diet high in magnesium-rich foods (see Power Tip below). But the most effective method of safely and effectively boosting your magnesium levels is through topical application onto your skin.

The fact that your body can absorb magnesium *transdermally* (through the skin) has been known for hundreds of years. Have you ever heard that taking a bath in Epsom salts was great for eliminating pain, reducing stress, and getting a good night's sleep? Epsom salt is actually a form of magnesium called magnesium sulfate.

Today, radically better forms of topical magnesium have been developed. Things like magnesium bath flakes and standard magnesium oils are usually 20 percent absorbable at best. The topical magnesium that I use and that I recommend for my clients is 100 percent bioavailable and 100 percent pure, and the stuff just flat-out works. A night hardly ever goes by that I don't rub this magnesium into my skin, because I've consistently found that my sleep quality is even better when I use it.

Again, because a large percentage of magnesium is lost in the digestive process, the ideal form of magnesium is transdermal from supercritical extracts. You can find more information on my favorite topical magnesium, Ease Magnesium, in the bonus resource guide at sleepsmarterbook.com/bonus.

◇ ◇ ◇ ◇

GOOD-SLEEP NUTRIENTS
POWER TIP #1

Keep the topical magnesium right by your bedside and apply it right before you hop under the covers. The best places to apply it are:

1. Anywhere that you are sore (hopefully you're following my exercise advice, covered in Chapter 11!)
2. In the center of your chest (a major position aligned with your heart— one of the most magnesium-dependent organs in your body—and your thymus gland—one of the major regulators of your immune system)
3. Around your neck and shoulders (where many people carry a lot of their stress)

Spray it on liberally and massage it in. Four to six sprays per area is a great baseline to go with.

GOOD-SLEEP NUTRIENTS
POWER TIP #2

Incorporate magnesium-rich foods in your diet, too. A study done by James Penland, PhD, at the Human Nutrition Research Center in Grand Forks,

North Dakota, found that a diet high in magnesium and low in aluminum was associated with deeper, uninterrupted sleep. Green leafy veggies, seeds like pumpkin and sesame, and superfoods like spirulina and Brazil nuts can provide very concentrated sources of magnesium for you.

GOOD-SLEEP NUTRIENTS
POWER TIP #3

There are several potential causes of constantly waking up in the middle of the night, but one commonly overlooked cause is trouble in the gastrointestinal tract, namely parasites. It's a big mistake to believe that parasites exist only in underdeveloped countries. They can definitely be more prevalent there, but parasites are everywhere. It's just the way that the planet works. These are opportunistic organisms that want to stow away in your belly and tissues and use you like public transportation with an all-you-can-eat buffet. Research has shown that parasites can make you outright sick, but they can also do things like influence food cravings and, according to *New York Times* bestselling author Amy Myers, MD, even upset your body's circadian rhythms and disrupt your sleep.

Parasites can be picked up through food, water, pets, unprotected sex, public toilet seats, and other ways as well. It's not something to freak out about because a strong immune system will help keep these organisms off and out of you. However, because so many people's health is already compromised today, getting a parasitic infection becomes that much easier. This is yet another reason why fortifying your immune system through eating more good-sleep nutrients (and more immuno-supportive nutrition overall) is so important to your health.

If you are consistently waking up at night, and you think parasites might be a problem, it's better to be safe than sorry and get it checked out. The problem is that standard forms of testing don't give extensive, accurate results. According to Dr. Myers, "The best way to test for a parasite is to get a stool test. Most doctors will run a conventional stool test if they suspect a parasite; however, these are not as accurate as the comprehensive stool tests that we use in functional medicine." You can find out how to get an accurate, comprehensive test done anywhere in the United States (as well as a few additional countries) by utilizing the information in the Sleep Smarter bonus resource guide. Be like Harrison Ford in the movie *Air Force One* and tell the stowaways, "Get off my plane!"

GOOD-SLEEP NUTRIENTS
POWER TIP #4

Do your best to avoid potentially gut-damaging chemicals that can hinder serotonin and melatonin production. Strive to eat organic, locally grown, unprocessed foods for the bulk of your diet. Leave some room for fun stuff, but make it a mandate that the vast majority of your foods are safe and nourishing to your gut health, brain, and sleep. Be sure to get in three to five servings of foods that contain the good-sleep nutrients above every day, and you'll be well on your way to improving your sleep from the inside out.

CHAPTER 8

CREATE A SLEEP SANCTUARY

If getting rejuvenating sleep is a high priority for you, then you need to take some essential actions to treat it as such. The bedroom should be for two things primarily . . . 1) sleep and 2) we'll get to in just a moment. ;-)

Humans are creatures of habit *and* habitat. The human brain is always looking for patterns so that it can automate behavior based on our environment. After a while, you don't have to consciously think about what you do when you go into different rooms in your home at certain times each day. You just go into those rooms, and you do them. It may be walking into the kitchen in the morning and flipping on the coffee maker; it might be strolling into the living room after work and turning on the TV; it might be stepping into the bathroom at night, grabbing your toothbrush, and brushing your teeth. You don't really have to put a lot of thought into these things; they just seem to happen. As a matter of fact, if you try to do them differently, they might even seem uncomfortable. (Have you ever tried brushing your teeth with the opposite hand? It can feel so awkward that you might as well be using your feet.)

Why do these behaviors become automated, and why is it so difficult to do something differently? To put it simply, this is how your brain is wired, and it's all thanks to the amazing power of something called *myelin*.

Myelin is a fatty material that coats, protects, and insulates nerves, enabling them to quickly conduct impulses between the brain and different parts of the body. Myelin wraps around nerve pathways (which control your activities), and it grows each time an action is repeated—making the signal move much faster and much more smoothly over time. This is what's responsible for what we often refer to as *muscle memory*.

The growth of myelin is what creates the difference between someone's first unusual swing at driving a golf ball—where they have to think about every little detail, and still only hit it half as far as they're capable of—versus years of swinging and being able to drive the ball great lengths without even worrying about the mechanics. Not everyone starts off hitting the ball hundreds of yards like Happy Gilmore, and the greatest golfers in the world have so automated the behavior that it comes just as naturally to them as breathing.

Neurons that fire together, wire together. So what you do repeatedly will, in fact, become a solid structure in your brain. When it comes to your sleeping environment, if you allow your bedroom to be a place where a lot of random activities take place, then you probably aren't creating a strong neuro-association to sleep when you go in there.

When you step into your bedroom, parts of your brain might light up expecting to watch television, or to break out the laptop for doing work, or answering e-mails, or scrolling through social media sites. Your brain is going to do what it's used to, not necessarily what you want it to do. You may think that you are a big "grown-up" adult and can make your own decisions about when to sleep, but we are all just super-size babies with the same basic programming. The environment you create in your bedroom, and the things you do in your bedroom, can have a significant impact on the quality of sleep you get.

One big takeaway point is that bringing your office work to bed with you can be one of the most offensive sleep crimes you can commit. Not only is it creating a negative association with sleep, but it can also spell serious trouble for your love life if you're not careful. We'll talk more about things to possibly extract from your bedroom to improve the quality of your sleep in Chapter 12. For now, let's focus on what small additions you can make to your bedroom to create a sleep sanctuary and get the best sleep possible.

BREATHE AGAIN

When you picture a sanctuary, what do you think of? Fresh air, flowing water, beautiful plants, and a serene environment may come to mind. The good news is that these are all things you can re-create in your own private sleep sanctuary.

Fresh air is very important. Did you know that the ions in the air you breathe can become "stale" and less energizing? The air you breathe carries more than just oxygen into your cells; it also carries other ionic elements that are vital for your health and well-being. As the air inside your home becomes stagnant, the ions in the air start to lose their (negative) charge. To fix this, you simply need to get the air moving again. Something as simple as opening a window or turning on a fan can re-energize the air in your bedroom.

If you are in a crazy situation where you don't have a window, or it's 20 below zero outside, you can use a high-quality air ionizer to revitalize the air in your home. Negative ions are present in abundance near waterfalls, ocean surf, rivers, and mountains. Many of us have experienced breathing the "fresh air" in those environments and experientially know the healing benefits. You can actually simulate some of those positive effects by utilizing the right air ionizer.

Negative ions improve our health in three significant ways:

1. They make the air more energizing by providing free electrons.
2. They oxidize odors, fungi, mold, parasites, and toxic chemical gases.
3. They bind to dust, pollen, cigarette smoke, and pet dander to form larger particles (which make them much easier to remove from your home).

Air ionizers are not just good for your sleeping space; they are good for your home in general. There are several air ionizers on the market, but you can find a list of my favorites in the bonus resource guide at sleepsmarterbook.com/bonus.

At a minimum, if you're in a situation where fresh air can't flow through your room via a window or fan during the winter months, try using a basic humidifier. Not only can this improve the air quality and help you sleep, but it can also help prevent your mucous membranes from drying out and making you more susceptible to an infection.

Humidifiers bring a bit of moisture back to the air, providing that water element we'd find in a sanctuary environment. In addition, some people find that the sounds of tabletop fountains or "mini-waterfalls" are great for relaxing and sleeping better at night. Obviously, I'm not talking about the drip from a leaky faucet, but studies show that both your heartbeat and breathing slow down after listening to running water. The sound of running water can actually have an impressive effect on people who have a history of sleep problems.

GARDEN OF EDEN

One of the things synonymous with paradise is plant life. There are so many great benefits that you can get from having plants in your home that it's just too much to ignore. Now, you don't have to have plants dominating your crib like in *Little Shop of Horrors*, but having an intelligently chosen houseplant or two can really do wonders.

Take the English ivy, for example. NASA listed it as the number one air-filtering houseplant. It has an unmatched ability to absorb formaldehyde (a known neurotoxin), which most of us are exposed to in our highly industrialized world today. It's incredibly easy to grow, and it's adaptable. You can have it as a hanging or a floor plant, and it requires moderate temperatures and medium sunlight.

Another great plant for your sleep sanctuary is the perennial snake plant. It doesn't require much light or water to thrive. What's most impressive about it is that it absorbs carbon dioxide and releases oxygen during the night (while most plants do this during the day), so it's the perfect plant to keep in your bedroom for a boost in air quality.

Not to be negated, the sight and *smell* of certain plants also have calming effects on the human body. Take the viney plant jasmine, for example. According to a study by the Wheeling Jesuit University in West Virginia, jasmine has a positive effect on the quality of sleep one gets, decreasing anxiety and improving the attitude one has after waking up. The smell of jasmine wasn't found to make people sleep more, but instead, to improve the *quality* of sleep by reducing interruptions in normal sleep patterns. Though jasmine hasn't been a traditional houseplant, it's now starting to grow in popularity. Additionally, the essential oils of jasmine and other plants have been shown to have many of the same positive effects. You can use an essential oil diffuser or simply dab a couple of drops right onto your pillowcase just before bed if you'd like to utilize the benefits that way.

Whether it's getting some plants, adding the soothing sound of water, or improving the air quality, do whatever it takes for *you* to feel relaxed and comfortable in your sleep sanctuary. Make your bedroom a sacred place where peace, calm, and relaxation are overflowing. Then, when you walk into your sleep sanctuary, it'll be easy to peacefully drift off to your dreams.

◇◇◇◇

SLEEP SANCTUARY
POWER TIP #1

Get at least one houseplant to improve the air quality in your home and go from there. If you don't have a green thumb and can barely take care of your own personal grooming (let alone a plant), then get a really low-maintenance plant, please. The pros of having a houseplant are simply too good to pass up; just make sure that it's something that suits you and not an additional stressor. If you don't have a good resource for houseplants, simply check out the options in the Sleep Smarter bonus resource guide to see where to find many of the most popular varieties (some can even be delivered right to your door).

SLEEP SANCTUARY
POWER TIP #2

If you share a sleeping space with someone else, make an agreement with them to keep office work out of the bedroom. This is a sacred space for both of you, and usually it just takes a heart-to-heart conversation to make sure that everyone is on the same page. The biggest person to hold to the agreement is yourself, so have the discipline to keep your bed reserved for sleep and what's coming up next in Chapter 9.

CHAPTER 9

HAVE A BIG "O"

This is the other primary thing that the bedroom should be used for (as if you didn't know). Having an orgasm can be like a full-on sedative for most people. Research shows that during orgasm, both women and men release a cocktail of chemicals, including oxytocin, serotonin, norepinephrine, vasopressin, and the pituitary hormone prolactin.

But, the proof is in the pudding, right? Even though most of us know that orgasm can induce sleep, are people actually using this to their advantage? Let's take a deeper look at this chemical cocktail to understand why sex can be so helpful for getting a great night's sleep.

OXYTOCIN

Oxytocin is sometimes referred to as the love hormone or the cuddle hormone because it promotes bonding between people when they're engaged in intimate activities like hugging, touching, and, of course, having sex.

Oxytocin levels are increased through orgasm, and according to research published in the journal *Regulatory Peptides*, oxytocin has a calming effect that counters the effects of cortisol and helps to promote sleep.

Oxytocin is normally produced in the hypothalamus and stored in the pituitary gland. With its deep connection to the major glands and organs in the body, its release also triggers a cascade of bodily events including the release of other feel-good chemicals called endorphins. This rush of relaxing hormones and endorphins when you release can be just the thing to set you up for great sleep. And a little fun fact about the word *endorphins*: It's derived from the words *endogenous* (produced from within) and *morphine*, from Morpheus, the god of sleep in Greek mythology.

SEROTONIN

Since we've discussed serotonin in previous chapters, you already know the tremendous influence that it has on your sleep. Sex is just another way you can instantly up your body's release of this powerful anti-stress neurotransmitter. Serotonin also flows when you feel significant or important, so it's not just about the sex; it's about the relationships, the connection, and the experience overall.

According to research published in the journal *Progress in Neurobiology*, serotonin is critical in obtaining and maintaining normal sleep-wake cycles, just like the adrenal-based hormone norepinephrine.

NOREPINEPHRINE

Also referred to as noradrenaline, norepinephrine functions in the human brain and body as a hormone and neurotransmitter. It has an important role in regulating your body's arousal system and maintaining normal states of sleep.

At the onset of sleep, serotonin is secreted, which increases deep, non-REM sleep. Secretion of norepinephrine takes place during REM sleep to help promote the efficacy of REM sleep and all of the physiological benefits that it provides. Research indicates that the fluctuation between these stages of sleep is largely due to the relationship between these two neurotransmitters.

Norepinephrine is also involved in the synthesis of melatonin, and it helps to regulate normal sleep-wake cycles that way as well. Released by the central nervous system, autonomic nervous system, and adrenals, norepinephrine plays a crucial part in balancing the overall stress response in the body.

VASOPRESSIN

A study published in the *Journal of Clinical Psychopharmacology* found that vasopressin increases sleep quality and decreases levels of cortisol in relationship to sleep.

Vasopressin is synthesized in the hypothalamus and stored in the posterior pituitary. Evidence suggests it plays an important role in social behavior, sexual motivation, pair bonding, and overall responses to stress. It's a fairly complex hormone with many functions, but the fact that it can be released directly into the brain after sex leads researchers to believe that it helps increase the relaxation response along with oxytocin.

PROLACTIN

Prolactin is a hormone that's linked to sexual satisfaction, and it's also heavily related to sleep. Studies show that prolactin levels are naturally higher during sleep, and animals injected with the chemical become tired immediately.

Studies clearly demonstrate that plasma prolactin concentrations are substantially increased for more than an hour following orgasm for both men and women. With that said, we can finally understand why sex is sometimes referred to as sleeping with someone.

Because prolactin is connected to sexual satisfaction, its release is the reason that men generally can't "go another round" and need time to recover. It's also important to note that men produce *four times* more prolactin when having an orgasm through intercourse as compared to masturbation.

For women, prolactin surges are deeply connected to the quality of orgasm and subsequent sexual satisfaction, according to research published in the *Journal of Sexual Medicine*. This pituitary hormone is associated with improved immune system function, great sleep, and improved quality of life. It's yet another reason to get a little closer and enjoy the health-giving benefits of the big "O."

DOING IT THE OTHER WAY

Not only does good sex lead to good sleep, but according to recent studies, good sleep also leads to good sex.

A study published in the *Journal of Sexual Medicine* found that women who got a more optimal amount of sleep had greater levels of sexual desire and greater arousal during sex. There was also found to be a 14 percent increase in the likelihood of sexual activity the next day after good sleep.

This should be a big note to the significant others out there: If you want a healthy, happy woman, then you have to do what you can to ensure that she gets great sleep at night.

Lack of sleep leads to lowered libido and poor sexual health in both sexes. Testosterone is a huge player in this, and data provided by the journal *Brain Research* found that sleep deprivation intrinsically leads to reduced testosterone in men. Low testosterone can give way to a whole host of issues such as increased storage of body fat, depression, and even erectile dysfunction.

According to Jon L. Pryor, MD, professor of urologic surgery at the University of Minnesota Medical School in Minneapolis, "Sleep deprivation can increase your risk of erectile dysfunction." This is because testosterone levels plummet when you don't get enough sleep. And to exacerbate the situation even more, you might not even care too much because low testosterone leads to low sexual desire.

To improve your sexual health, it is a must that you improve your sleep. This is one of the force multipliers that people commonly look past in efforts to regain their vitality, energy, and desire. Lack of sleep can make things exponentially worse, and high-quality sleep can make things exponentially better.

PRACTICING SAFE SLEEP

Sex and orgasm have many benefits that go far beyond the realm of sleep, from boosting the immune system, to fighting depression, to actually helping you to live a longer life. Our ability to have and give orgasms is tightly linked to our health and well-being.

And just to be clear again on why this is so effective, the brain is actually the largest sex organ because of the vital role it plays in sexual arousal (whoever said size doesn't matter?). Cultivating your brain-body connection is critical to a fulfilling sex life *and* getting the best sleep ever.

Be responsible, have fun, and enjoy the benefits that the big "O" can add to your life.

◇ ◇ ◇ ◇

THE BIG "O"
POWER TIP #1

Communication is always the key in this area. Everyone is different, and what satisfies one person might not do a thing for another. Find out what your lover likes and find out what *you* like. Share this info with them because being a clairvoyant is not on most of our résumés.

Share with your partner what turns you on, and what takes you over the top. I promise you that this data will be valuable to you both.

THE BIG "O"
POWER TIP #2

Nutrition and exercise are also a critical part of supporting your sexual health. Be sure to include plenty of the *good-sleep nutrients* and foods from Chapter 7 in your diet every day (as most of them are proven to support the reproductive system, too!). There will be more powerhouse nutrition and exercise information coming up in later chapters, so be ready to take action on it, and you'll soon see the results for yourself.

THE BIG "O"
POWER TIP #3

Get physical. An obvious aspect of sex's impact on sleep is the physical exertion involved. When you put in some work bumpin' and grindin', you'll naturally feel more fatigued after the session is over. You don't have to just lie there most of the time all vanilla-ice-cream style. Move around, get involved, and put your back into it. Lying back and receiving is super fine as well, but if you want to earn your sleep black belt, then you've got to put some work in, too.

CHAPTER 10

GET IT BLACKED OUT

It's a well-established fact that we sleep better in a dark environment, yet so many people aren't taking full advantage of this.

Having light sources of any type in your bedroom can disrupt your sleep patterns. And even using an eye mask is not going to be 100 percent effective for most people.

Did you know that your skin actually has receptors that can pick up light? These photoreceptors are similar to those found in your retina, so your skin can *literally* see. Researchers at Brown University discovered that skin cells also make *rhodopsin*, a light-sensitive chemical found in the retina. If there's light in your bedroom, your body is picking it up and sending messages to your brain and organs that can interfere with your sleep.

One study conducted at Cornell University took action to test this out. The researchers put a fiber-optic cable behind the knee of a test subject and illuminated a patch of skin that was no bigger than the size of a quarter. Even though the subject slept in what was otherwise complete darkness, that small amount of light was enough to affect the subject's body temperature and melatonin secretion. This reiterates the point that it's not just about covering your eyes; it's about creating a sleep environment that helps bring about the best sleep possible.

THE DARK SIDE OF LIGHT

Sleeping in total darkness is so significant that nighttime light has been dubbed "light pollution." Light pollution refers to any adverse effects from artificial light. Humans (and most other organisms for that matter) evolved to adjust to predictable light and dark phases to set their circadian clocks. Once artificial light became the societal norm, it effectively changed the length of our days. Instead of a 12-hour day, we can now artificially create a 24-hour day with nonstop light exposure. Though research indicates that some ancient human civilizations slept a similar amount of hours as our society today, it's the *quality* of sleep that's so drastically different. Our natural light and dark cycles are being disrupted, and our sleep is suffering as a result.

One of the most devastating impacts of this light pollution is the confirmed effect on melatonin production. Studies show that exposure to room light during usual hours of sleep suppresses melatonin levels by more than 50 percent. That's not good!

We've already discussed how valuable melatonin is for sleep, but there are many other things that it supports in your body. Melatonin has been proven to:

- Improve immune system function
- Normalize blood pressure
- Reduce the proliferation of cancer cells and tumor growth (including leukemia)
- Enhance DNA protection and free radical scavenging
- Decrease risk of osteoporosis
- Decrease risk of plaques in the brain (like those seen with Alzheimer's disease)
- Alleviate migraines and other pain
- Improve thyroid function
- Improve insulin sensitivity and weight reduction

Melatonin is like the Bo Jackson of hormones. If it has something to do with health, melatonin "knows" how to help.

Not getting enough sleep, and not sleeping in darkness, will age you faster and suck away your vitality. So, with all the newfound data to back it up, the best solution for improving your sleep is to get your room blacked out.

Get yourself some of the now popular "blackout" curtains that are available from most retailers. And get any other sources of nonstop light out of your bedroom as well. Do these two things tonight, and I promise you that you'll thank me for it tomorrow. Sleep experts suggest that your room be so dark that you can't see your hand in front of your face. I grew up with nightlights, so this was a really big step for me, too.

Speaking of nightlights, researchers from the Scheie Eye Institute at the University of Pennsylvania in Philadelphia discovered that even a simple nightlight could contribute to myopia in children and lead to significant vision problems later in life. In the study, 479 children under the age of 2 were put into one of three categories: Sleeps in a) total darkness, b) with a nightlight on, or c) with a room light on. The results were shocking.

The researchers found that 10 percent of children who slept in the dark ended up being nearsighted, while 34 percent of the children who slept with a nightlight and 55 percent of the children who slept in a lightened room developed nearsightedness. Though the study didn't account for every variable possible, it's definitely something to consider. This isn't just important for us as adults; it's also important if you have children and grandchildren.

Sleeping in total darkness is something that our genes expect us to do. Today it's not uncommon to have lights of some type beaming in your room all night long. Because you can't control the world outside, you need to take full control of the world in your home. New headlights and street lamps that use LEDs emit some of the most sleep-zapping light spectrums of all. This is why getting some blackout shades is so significant.

Take action to turn your bedroom into a nice, cozy sleep cave. Personally, this is the one thing that *instantly* had a beneficial impact on my sleep. I blacked out my bedroom and have been getting the best sleep of my life ever since.

LUX CAPACITOR

Since we can't go back in time and change the fact that our society has become so dependent on light, there are a couple of things you can do to reduce the burden that excessive light can have on your body.

A study at Harvard Medical School found that exposure to light at night throws the body's biological clock out of whack, which you already know. But what they also discovered was that not all colors of light have the same effect.

The Harvard researchers conducted an experiment comparing the effects of 6½ hours of exposure to blue light (like you get from the screens of our everyday tech devices) to exposure to green light of comparable brightness. The blue light suppressed melatonin for about twice as long as the green light did and shifted circadian rhythms by twice as much (3 hours versus 1½ hours).

The research indicates that just by changing the color spectrum of light you're exposed to at night, you can help prevent melatonin from being bullied by the Biff-like power of blue lighting.

Colors even have a correlating temperature that influences their impact on the human body. According to the Kelvin scale, blue light is at the farthest end of the spectrum, meaning it occurs at higher temperatures, while red occurs at lower, cooler temperatures. This is the opposite of the cultural associations attributed to colors in which red is "hot" and blue is "cold."

This explains why Harvard researchers recommend using dim red lights at night. According to their data, "Red light has the *least* power to shift circadian rhythm and suppress melatonin."

ILLUMINANCE PROVIDED UNDER VARIOUS CONDITIONS

ILLUMINANCE	SURFACES ILLUMINATED BY:
0.0001 lux	Moonless, overcast night sky (starlight)
0.002 lux	Moonless clear night sky with airglow
0.27 to 1.0 lux	Full moon on a clear night
3.4 lux	Dark limit of civil twilight under a clear sky
50 lux	Family living room lights
80 lux	Office building hallway/toilet lighting
100 lux	Very dark overcast day
320 to 500 lux	Office lighting
400 lux	Sunrise or sunset on a clear day
1000 lux	Overcast day; typical TV studio lighting
10,000 to 25,000 lux	Full daylight (not direct sun)
32,000 to 100,000 lux	Direct sunlight

Instead of basking in the hot light of standard bulbs from our lamps and overhead lights, try utilizing the soft light of candles in the evening to transition to a great night of sleep. Humans have been using the cherished glow of fire for eons to cook our food, warm our bodies, and light our way at night. But remember, it's still a tiny fire being lit in your home, so use candles with respect and attentiveness.

You can even swap out certain lights in your home or a couple of lamps with red bulbs. It might assist in setting a sexy mood to help out with what you learned in Chapter 9. Whether you are a fan of rock 'n' roll, R & B, country, or even K-pop, the influence of red light is enough to have quite a few songs written about it.

It's still helpful to remember that it's not just about the color of light (though that is extremely important); it's also about the luminance. Lux is the unit used to measure luminance. As you can see from the chart, the lux from direct sunlight is upwards of 100,000. Compare that with the normal light exposure our ancestors would get from moonlight (at under 1 tiny lux), and you can see how abnormal our typical evening light exposure can be.

Indoor lighting can range from 50 to 500 lux, automatically triggering a suppression of melatonin if you're unprotected from these lights at night. Follow the recommendations in Chapter 3 for lessening your screen exposure after dark, utilize cooler-color lights at home in the evening, and take action to get your bedroom as dark as possible at night to ensure you get the melatonin production and sleep that you really need.

◇ ◇ ◇ ◇

GET IT BLACKED OUT
POWER TIP #1

You don't just want to block out the light from outside; you want to eliminate the troublesome light inside your bedroom, too. One of the biggest culprits is that angry alarm clock staring at you. The alarm clocks with the white or blue digits are more disruptive than ones with red digits. You can start by simply covering the alarm clock up as one tactic. Another option is to find a digital alarm clock with a dimmer adjustment that allows you to turn the clock light all the way off. Cover the clock up or get a better clock—either way, you'll be doing yourself a favor.

GET IT BLACKED OUT
POWER TIP #2

In preparation for sleeping in your pitch-black room, lowering the luminosity of the lights in your home (turning down the lights) or utilizing different color bulbs is a very good idea. As the data shows, red lights are great, plus candle light can be a nice alternative. Additionally, Himalayan salt lamps feature a soft pinkish-orange tint. Some research indicates that salt lamps can produce a small amount of the health-giving negative ions that we talked about in Chapter 8. So this goes to show that you don't have to really love tie-dyed shirts in order to enjoy a salt lamp.

GET IT BLACKED OUT
POWER TIP #3

The purpose of using blackout curtains is really to block out unnatural light that would be making its way into your home. But if you live in an area where you don't have street lights, a neighbor's porch light, or cars constantly driving up and down your road, then getting blackout curtains is not totally necessary. Sure, you might have some illuminating moonlight during certain times of the month, but as you can see on the lux chart, moonlight is only a fraction of a percent of what you'd be hit with from any other type of light. The caution over light pollution has more to do with unnatural light, not the natural light you'd get from the moon subtly reflecting the rays of the sun.

GET IT BLACKED OUT
POWER TIP #4

Once you have your blackout curtains, you may find that there is still some light that sneaks in over the top. You can simply roll up a blanket or towel to cover up that area. Physician and *New York Times* bestselling author Joseph Mercola, DO, recommends that, even during the midday sun, your bedroom should be very dark when you go in there. There shouldn't be any light sneaking in unless you want it to. Getting rid of the light pollution in your bedroom is a huge key to getting the most peaceful and rejuvenating sleep possible.

CHAPTER 11

TRAIN HARD (BUT SMART)

Exercise is often considered a virtual fountain of youth if used in the right way. Muscle, for example, is a reservoir for anti-aging hormones that help to protect your DNA from oxidation. The research shows that you can stay younger, longer if you have more lean muscle on your body.

How does exercise relate to sleep? Well, the two go together like peanut butter and jelly. You actually don't get in shape at the gym while you're exercising. You're literally tearing down your body while working out and creating thousands of tiny micro-tears in your muscle fibers. When you leave the gym, you're actually in *worse* shape than when you came in. If I were to take you in for blood work and a hormone panel after a great workout session, your stress hormones would be elevated, your inflammatory biomarkers would be up, and even your blood sugar would be a little abnormal. But there is nothing "wrong" with you. You just did a great workout that's going to do a lot of good for your body once it gets a chance to heal.

The secret is that your body is transformed from your workout while you sleep. This is when your body releases large amounts of beneficial hormones and elicits repair programs to build you up better than before. You just exposed yourself to a significant healthy stressor with a workout, but you only get the full reward if you properly rest and recover.

The big issue for many people is that they are turning this healthy stressor into an unhealthy stressor. Add exercise to the already big list of work issues, family issues, unpaid bills, poor diet, mental and emotional struggles, etc., and this creates what's known as your overall *stress load*.

Your stress load is the compilation of stress in your life. Stress doesn't have to be bad, but when you put yourself under too much of it, you can break down.

Exercise can be amazing for you. As a matter of fact, it's essential to being the healthiest version of yourself. You get so many positive benefits, from improving insulin sensitivity, to boosting healthy hormone function, to enhancing your metabolism. But when it's placed on top of an already overwhelming stress load, it can lead to some significant problems.

It's not so much the exercise itself, but the when and how the exercise is done. To optimize your sleep (and thus, optimize your results from exercise), you have to utilize a few principles when it comes to working out.

NIGHTTIME IS NOT THE RIGHT TIME

A recent study at Appalachian State University in Boone, North Carolina, found that morning workouts are ideal if you want to get the best sleep at night. Researchers tracked the sleep patterns of participants who worked out at three different times: 7:00 a.m., 1:00 p.m., or 7:00 p.m.

What they discovered was that people who exercised at 7:00 a.m. slept longer and had a deeper sleep cycle than the other two groups. In fact, the morning exercisers had up to 75 percent more time in the reparative "deep sleep" stage at night. This is so impressive, and a huge leverage point if you're interested in a longer life and a better body.

This may be counterintuitive for people who believe that you can fall asleep faster after going through a tough workout. One of the big issues with working out late in the evening is that it significantly raises your core body temperature, and it can take upwards of 4 to 6 hours for your temperature to come down again. As we discussed in Chapter 5, your body goes through a process of thermoregulation to lower your core temperature to create the optimal environment for sleep. By aimlessly raising your core temperature with a workout too close to bedtime you can prevent yourself from getting the best sleep possible.

But, no need to be worried if you choose to work out a little later in the day. It's been found that when your core temperature comes down after exercise, it actually goes a little bit lower than it normally would. So, if you time things up intelligently, this can be money when it comes to getting the best sleep.

Exercising in the late afternoon or early evening is a great idea from a thermoregulation perspective. If you work out at 4:30 p.m., for example, it can set you up nicely to hit the hay at 10:00 p.m. By then, the stress hormones secreted from your workout have subsided, your parasympathetic nervous system (the "rest and digest" system) has had time to take over, and your core temperature has dropped down to set the optimal internal environment for sleepy time.

So, if you have to pick a time to work out, morning is the best when it comes to sleep, early evening can provide some benefit (if you time things right), and smack-dab in the afternoon shows little to no benefit at all as far as blatant sleep benefits are concerned. Exercise and movement is important no matter when you do it, but we have natural hormonal cycles that we need to honor if we're going to get the most from it.

As you know from the cortisol release chart in Chapter 2, we have a big spike of cortisol in the early morning that is for the sole purpose of doing activity. This is precisely why morning exercise is so helpful for improving your sleep. It can help to encourage that normal release of cortisol in the morning and put your cortisol cycle right on track. From there, it gradually drops during the day and bottoms out when it's our natural time to get to sleep. This is why working out at 1 o'clock in the morning is cute for a Facebook status to show your dedication, but it's plumb dumb when it comes to protecting your mind and body from the deleterious effects of stress.

Today it's pretty common to see 24-hour gyms with dedicated people working out late into the night. I've been a willing participant in late night exercise many times myself. (Note: This was in college while my decision-making skills weren't fully developed.) I would head down to the gym and train after 10:00 p.m., play competitive midnight basketball, or even go for a late night run or two.

When we are younger, we tend to participate in behaviors like these and not think anything of it. Many of us can eat whatever crazy foods we want, stay up late until the wee hours of the morning, and still be able to get up and pass our exams. Just 10 years later, if you try to pull that stuff, you likely feel like a certified mess.

Well, what happened? Why could so many of us eat things like double stuffed crust pizza all the time when we were younger and still stay relatively lean? Why could we stay up late (knowing all of the harmful effects you know now) and still be able to function? Well, to put it simply, at that time in our lives we have the hormones of a mythical beast (not a scientific term, but it fits rather nicely). We are just churning out anabolic hormones that are trying to help propel our gene pool to be successful in the future.

This is why all of us look so different when we compare our pictures from when we were 6, 16, and whatever age you're at now. Your body changed because your hormones changed. And this is where the real transformational power is located. We'll talk more about optimizing your hormone function and getting some of that youthful juice (aka mythical beast juice) back in your system in Chapter 13. For now it's critical to understand that those behaviors in your college days aren't without a cost. As a matter of fact, the research shows that those behaviors actually accelerate your aging and speed up the date that your youth and vitality slip out of your hand.

TONIGHT WE ARE YOUNG—TOMORROW, NOT SO MUCH

The most accurate biological markers we have that can tell us how long we're going to live are something called *telomeres*. Telomeres are like the little plastic end caps on the tips of your shoestrings that keep them from fraying. But instead of it being your shoestrings, telomeres are the end caps on your chromosomes that keep *them* from breaking down and fraying.

As we age, segments of our telomeres get clipped off until eventually there is nothing left and there's a breakdown of the cellular material. In rudimentary terms, this is what aging looks like. It happens every day, but slowly over the years, though there is one big issue: It's been confirmed that certain lifestyle practices can either slow down or accelerate the loss of your telomere length. Research conducted by scientists at the University of California found that sleep deprivation is one of the single biggest triggers for accelerated loss of your telomere length.

What this means is that those days in our teens and early twenties when we decided to forgo the sleep our bodies need, we could definitely "get by" easier, but we're unknowingly accelerating our aging so much that we won't even know what hit us when it all suddenly stops.

Suddenly you don't have the energy you once did; suddenly you get sick more often; suddenly you start to experience more aches and pains; suddenly it's incredibly difficult to get rid of unwanted weight. I'm not talking about people in their seventies and eighties—I'm talking about millions of people experiencing this in their late twenties! We're inadvertently speeding up our aging process and hardly anyone has the opportunity to figure out why.

This is the reason it's essential that this information about sleeping smarter is shared readily with our kids—especially high school and college students—so that they can be armed with the knowledge that's going to support them in staying healthy, strong, and youthful for many years to come.

The good news for all of us is that our telomere length can be fortified with healthy lifestyle factors. Research published in *Archives of Internal Medicine* found that people who did a moderate amount of exercise—about 100 minutes a week of activity such as tennis, swimming, or running—had telomeres that on average looked like those of someone about 5 or 6 years younger as compared to those who did the least exercise—about 16 minutes a week. This reiterates the fact that exercise can be like an all-you-can-drink fountain of youth. Couple that with the improvements it delivers for your sleep, and you can see why smart exercise is a must for our health and longevity.

The big key here is to time your exercise appropriately. Clearly, staying up late has its downside, but exercising late has an even bigger downside. And it's not just about staying up late and working out in the evening; it's also not a good idea to interrupt your sleep to get up at 3:00 a.m. to go trudge along on the treadmill. Your natural hormone cycles are not designed to be up at those hours going hard in the gym. Take full advantage of this knowledge and structure your life in a way that allows you to exercise at the best time to have the body and health you deserve. You have more power in this than you think. Remember, we are not just products of our environment; we are *creators* of our environment!

INSANE IN THE MEMBRANE

I had a client a few years back who moved here to the United States from France to go to college. He came to work with me in the gym and had some very specific physical goals that he wanted to accomplish. After doing an analysis, I found out that he had been suffering from a sleeping disorder for about 8 years. He typically didn't sleep for more than 4 hours a night, and he was diagnosed with clinical insomnia.

I can tell you, it was written all over his face and body. I said to him, "I can kick your butt all day in the gym, but you'll never get the body you want until you get this sleep component in order." He was reluctant to focus on it because it had been so difficult for him in the past, but he agreed to try a few of my suggestions, and the rest was, as the French say, *histoire.*

Instead of the long-duration cardio he used to do, I *banned* him from cardio temporarily. We focused on heavy, superset-style strength training. His workouts were short, but intense, and within days everything changed.

He came in to see me about a week after he started training with me and said, "I don't know what you did, but I slept like a bébé" (remember, it was a French accent). This was quite transformative for him, and his life was changed forever.

Again, exercise is a stressor in and of itself. It's known as a *hormetic* stressor—something that, in the right dose, can be incredibly beneficial to the human body. But that's true if, and only if, your body is allowed to adapt (i.e., get the sleep you need).

Conventional moderate-pace jogging is the mother of all long-duration catabolic exercise. You're keeping your sympathetic nervous system firing continuously for the 30 minutes or so that you're jogging, plus all of the stress hormones you secrete don't get a chance to be broken down and eliminated—they build up in your body like a balloon being filled with too much water.

Can running be good for you? Absolutely. But it comes with some important caveats. We've been misled to believe that "cardio" in the form of jogging for long time periods is the ideal way to lose fat. The reality is that nothing could be further from the truth. Running for long distances can radically increase muscle loss through a process called *gluconeogenesis.* Muscle is your body's fat-burning machinery, and if you lose it by running too much, you will depress your metabolism and find that if you don't keep running day after day, you'll start getting fat very quickly. You and Forrest Gump can keep on running, but I'm going to go ahead and sit this one out. Bottom line: You don't need to run for long time periods to lose fat. Thinking that is like thinking the tooth fairy exists.

The *biggest* caveat is that you should do long-distance running only if you truly love it. If the purpose of your running is not for fat loss, but instead, it's meditative and something that you just enjoy, then go for it! Just be aware and be smart about it, and make sure that you do some of the other stuff you're about to learn.

QUALITY OVER QUANTITY

To get the best hormonal response, you need to lift heavy weights. This will trigger your body to secrete more anabolic hormones that will enable you to feel better, look better, and sleep better.

Most men have no issues with this, but many women still have the idea that lifting heavy weights will make them "bulky." The reality is that most men who lift weights like crazy *still* struggle to put on size. Compared to women, men naturally have significantly higher levels of testosterone that aid in mass building, yet even that doesn't help them pack on the size just because they start weight training. Today's modern man will often resort to weight gain shakes, "dirty bulking" (aka eating a bunch of high-calorie crappy food), and tons of supplements—yet still see only lackluster results in getting bigger. So, unless a woman is taking a steroid cocktail and eating like it's her full-time job, she doesn't have to worry much at all about getting bulky. This is not what lifting heavy weight is about anyway. And I don't want a single woman to lose sight of the real unrivaled benefit that lifting weights can give you.

As a matter of fact, if you lose weight through the traditional ways of dieting and cardio, you'll simply be able to go from an apple shape to a smaller apple shape. By lifting weights, you can actually change your body's *composition* and potentially go from an apple shape to an hourglass shape. Lifting weights enables you to express your true genetic potential. Your genes expect you to lift heavy things, and when you do that, your body changes accordingly.

Bottom line: Lifting weights doesn't make you big; eating a large amount of food makes you big. Lifting weights won't make you big and bulky; chocolate croissants will make you big and bulky. (I'm still in my French state of mind right now.)

To optimize my former insomniac client's sleep, I had him lift weights for just three 30-minute sessions per week. He dropped body fat, improved his health biomarkers, and, most important, got the sleep he really required.

SLEEP, EXERCISE, EAT, REPEAT

Always remember that making regular exercise a part of your life isn't just about having a great body; it's about having great sleep. A study published in the *Journal of Clinical Sleep Medicine* found that patients with primary insomnia had a *radical* improvement in sleep quality when they added in a consistent exercise regimen.

The study used a *polysomnogram* to measure the results. A polysomnogram is a sleep test that records your brain waves, the oxygen level in your blood, heart rate, and breathing, as well as eye and leg movements (basically, there are so many wires on you while you sleep that it looks like Spider Man hit you with a web). Here's exactly what they discovered.

Test subjects who started exercising experienced:

- A 55 percent improvement in sleep onset latency (they fell asleep faster)
- A 30 percent decrease in the total wake time during the test
- An 18 percent increase in total sleep time during the test
- A 13 percent increase in sleep efficiency (an improvement in the quality of sleep)

All of this from adding in exercise. Not a pill. Not rubbing a magic lamp. But from exercise.

Studies show that there are improvements immediately, but the substantial benefit to sleep health kicks in after a couple weeks of consistent exercise. The key word here is *consistent*, and trying to create consistency after years of inconsistency can be like trying to herd cats.

It takes a smart approach and some specific triggers to ensure that exercise is a regular part of your life. I'm going to share some important insights with you in the Power Tips section to ensure that you exercise regularly and take the best possible care of yourself.

SLEEP AND ATHLETIC PERFORMANCE

It's not surprising that world-class athletes utilize sleep as a part of their overall training programs. Athletes like LeBron James, Roger Federer, and Michelle Wie average more than 10 hours of sleep per night. Venus Williams, Lindsey Vonn, and Usain Bolt hardly go a day without getting at least 8. Fatigue Science gathered statements from some of the top athletes on the planet, and Usain Bolt (the fastest man in history) said, "Sleep is extremely important to me—I need to rest and recover in order for the training I do to be absorbed by my body."

This quote perfectly states how your body doesn't change from the training alone; it changes based on the quality of sleep that you get.

Researchers at Stanford University actually set out to examine the benefits of sleep on athletic performance. The test subjects were members of the men's varsity basketball team, and the results they saw were absolutely shocking.

After increasing the amount of sleep they got (with the average ending up at $8\frac{1}{2}$ hours), board-certified sleep specialist Michael J. Breus, PhD, laid the data out like this:

- The athletes ran significantly faster: Players shaved nearly 1 full second off of their sprint times.
- Their shooting improved dramatically: Players saw their free-throw shooting and their three-point shooting improve by 9 percent.
- They felt less fatigue and less daytime sleepiness (and improved their reaction times as well).
- They reported an improvement in their moods and their overall physical well-being (during both games and practice).

If you want to perform at your best, then getting great sleep is an absolute must. It's a competitive advantage that we all have access to if we choose it and structure our time wisely. Remember, it's not just about sleeping more; it's about *sleeping smarter,* and the tips below are going to help you do just that.

◇ ◇ ◇ ◇

TRAIN SMART
POWER TIP #1

Whether you choose to do a full workout in the morning or afternoon, make sure to get some activity in during the first part of the day regardless. You don't have to hit the gym to encourage that natural hormone spike that helps to set you up for great sleep at night. You can take just a few minutes to do some body weight exercises, go for a power walk, do some rebounding on a mini-trampoline, do some yoga, hit a few sets of kettle bell swings, do Tabata, or so many other things. Doing just a few minutes of any of these won't interfere with your training later in the day (if that's when you choose to train).

If you prefer to do a full workout in the morning, then simply do that. Whatever way you slice it, the clinically proven benefits of activity in the morning are just too good to pass up.

TRAIN SMART
POWER TIP #2

Take out a schedule and block off specific appointment times for you to work out using the info above. You can set a time for the morning or early evening; just ensure that you're giving yourself the best advantage for getting great sleep. If you're really serious about being the healthiest person you can be, you'll set your personal exercise appointment and sleep time first, then schedule everything else around them.

TRAIN SMART
POWER TIP #3

Do something you enjoy! The best form of exercise is the exercise you'll actually do. It's difficult enough to fit exercise in with all of the things we have going on today. Why make it harder by planning to do something you don't like?

Strength training is obviously important for everybody based on what you've already learned, but there are many ways to go about getting the exercise you need and making it fun. Outside of a couple days of strength training (which is *essential*—and many people love doing this already), add some days of additional activities that you enjoy. Maybe it's basketball, maybe it's dancing, maybe yoga or Pilates classes. Whatever it may be for you, make a commitment to yourself to do that. You have a right to enjoy the process of getting well. Find something you love to do, and do it often.

TRAIN SMART
POWER TIP #4

Get an accountability partner. Statistics show that having external accountability drastically increases your rate of follow-through. When it comes to accountability, the most important prerequisite is to have a person (or people) who believes in you. It's not the best idea to look for support in people who might doubt you and shut you down (even unintentionally).

When you are working to change your body and your health, everyone around you might not be supportive. That's why it's so important to connect with people who are on the same path as you. I highly recommend listening to my number one rated health and fitness show (now downloaded in more than 180 countries!) to get the additional motivation, education, and empowering messages you need to help you get to a whole new level. Visit themodelhealthshow.com or subscribe to *The Model Health Show* on iTunes, Stitcher, or anywhere you can listen to podcasts on your favorite device. You can also join the Sleep Smarter Facebook group via the bonus resource guide (sleepsmarterbook.com/bonus) and get matched up with some helpful accountability there, too.

When selecting a one-on-one accountability partner, avoid choosing someone who has a history of struggling with the same challenge that you have. If your issue is simply getting to the gym, then don't partner up with someone else who struggles to get to the gym. That's like getting guidance on cooking from someone who barely knows their way around a microwave. Instead, look for someone who's better (at least a little bit) in the area that you need improvement in, and hopefully you can offer them the same in another area. That's how great partnerships and one-on-one accountability partners work.

TRAIN SMART
POWER TIP #5

It's not only that exercise impacts your sleep, but sleep also impacts your exercise. Research published in the *Journal of Clinical Sleep Medicine* found that a poor night's sleep led to less frequent and shorter workouts the next day.

The researchers set out to find if exercise improved sleep quality for insomniacs (which it did), but they were surprised to learn that if a night of poor sleep occurred, the next day the motivation to exercise would drop. It wasn't until after weeks of pushing through that better sleep and consistent exercise evened out. It's important to be aware of this and know that getting good sleep is a part of your overall motivation. But in the beginning, if you have to push yourself a little more to exercise, have the courage to do so, knowing that eventually you won't have to *push* because the vision of a better life and the way you feel will start to *pull* you.

TRAIN SMART
POWER TIP #6

Make sure that you're lifting weights at least 2 days per week. Focus on compound lifts that really give you the most bang for your buck. You can grab some sample step-by-step exercise protocols in the Sleep Smarter bonus resource guide. There are also free tips on how to line up your nutrition and supplementation (like how to strategically utilize caffeine) to accelerate fat loss from your workouts.

Even though the bonus resource guide is amazing, a little planning and common sense here will do just fine. If you have a history of sleep problems, I recommend short "superset" training sessions that last no longer than 30 minutes. You can do this by pairing two exercises together for noncompeting muscle groups. We'll use legs and chest in this example. Do 8 to 10 reps of weighted squats followed immediately by 8 to 10 reps of incline presses. Rest until fully recovered (upwards of 2 minutes), then repeat the superset again. You can switch up the exercises and rest time, but the basic format remains the same. Structuring your program like this is great for fat loss *and* optimizing your hormones for a better night's sleep.

CHAPTER 12

GET YOUR "FRIENDS" OUT OF YOUR ROOM

Cell phones, televisions, desktops, laptops, iPads, Kindles, tablets, and more. Many people have turned their bedrooms into miniature Best Buy locations. But what are the health risks associated with this? And what in the world is it doing to our sleep?

A study sponsored by mobile companies themselves found that talking on cell phones before bed caused people to take longer to reach critical deep stages of sleep *and* they spent less time in deep sleep. This translates to a diminished ability for the body to heal, depressed immune function, depressed hormone function, and poorer performance the following day.

Researchers at Loughborough University Sleep Research Centre in Leicestershire, England, set out to test the impact of cell phone radiation on the human brain. In the study, they strapped cell phones to the heads of study participants and monitored their brain waves by EEG while the phone was switched on and off by remote computer.

The experiment revealed that after the phone was switched to "talk" mode (as if you were on a call), brain wave patterns called delta waves remained depressed for more than 1 hour after the phone was turned off. These delta brain waves are the most reliable marker of deep sleep. A significant portion of your sleep consists of this stage, and interference with it will have a noticeable effect on sleep efficiency, which is exactly what the researchers observed.

When the test subjects were allowed to go to sleep, they ended up remaining awake twice as long after the phone was shut off. They could not fall into deeper levels of sleep for nearly 1 *full hour* after the cell phone radiation stopped playing hide-and-go-seek with their brain waves.

This is not a futile plea to break out the tin foil hats and hide from technology. As we know, our development and use of technology is ever expanding and a valuable part of our lives. However, it's a great idea to be aware of these potential issues and utilize smart strategies to protect ourselves accordingly.

The most alarming part is that right now at least 50 percent of Americans sleep with their cell phones right by their sides. Many people will admit to checking message alerts in the middle of the night (and needlessly disrupting their sleep patterns). Plus, many more will admit that the first thing they do is reach for their cell phone as soon as they wake up each day.

Our attention is enormously valuable, and how you begin and end your day has a huge impact on the results in your life. Starting the day checking e-mails and messages on your phone *immediately* puts other people's priorities ahead of yours. You start the day addressing other people's needs instead of taking time to care for yourself physically and getting focused on your own goals for the day. You are, in essence, saying, "I know I have things that I want to accomplish, but I would much rather try to take care of them last when I'm stressed out, out of time, and out of energy."

Ending your day by kissing your cell phone goodnight and laying it by your side is another surefire way to set yourself up for failure. Your thoughts are lingering on your last interaction on your phone and not your goals. And as we discussed in Chapter 3, the spectrum of light emitted from your cell phone screen triggers your brain to secrete more "daytime hormones," which delays and reduces the secretion of the sleepy-time hormone melatonin.

COOKING UP CANCER

We already covered some powerful reasons to keep your cell phone out of your bedroom, but the issues go far deeper than that. Our appliances and electronic devices emit both electric and magnetic fields known as EMFs. Electric fields are easily blocked by walls and other objects, but magnetic fields can pass through walls, buildings, and the human body with ease. EMFs have been found to cause disruption in the communication among the cells in our bodies.

Take a look at these two words and tell me what the difference is:

EAT FAT

If you have a keen eye, you'll notice that the only difference is the *one line* at the bottom of the "E." One line, one piece of data, caused an entirely different end result. Cellular communication within the body is just like this. If the wrong information is communicated among the upwards of 100 trillion cells you have, autoimmune diseases can manifest, hormones can be thrown out of whack, and even cancer cells can show their ugly faces.

EMFs from our common electronic friends have been linked to leukemia, brain tumors, and breast cancer, along with several other serious issues. So, what about cell phone EMFs?

The World Health Organization has now classified cell phone radiation as a Group 2B carcinogen.

Research author Siegal Sadetzki, MD, MPH, a cancer specialist at Tel Aviv University in Israel, testified at a US Senate hearing that cell phones were identified as a contributor to salivary gland tumors. The report states that your risk of getting a parotid tumor on the same side of your head that you use for listening to the cell phone increases by:

- 34 percent if you are a regular cell phone user and have used a mobile phone for 5 years
- 58 percent if you had more than about 5,500 calls in your lifetime
- 49 percent if you have spoken on the phone for more than 266.3 hours during your lifetime

Still not convinced?

A study published in *Radiation Protection Dosimetry* found that melatonin secretion is significantly disrupted by exposure to electromagnetic fields. The study's authors concluded that it would be in our best interest if we limit our exposure even to weak EMFs. As you know, melatonin is not just a critical hormone for regulating our sleep; it's also an important anti-cancer hormone. With consistent exposure to EMFs, our body's melatonin production can be thrown out of whack.

It's important to realize that WiFi and various forms of radio waves are extremely new forms of energy that we humans have been playing around with. We know that the human body is extremely conductive, and because it has been such a short time since we've had this form of technology, we still don't know the long-term impact of creating a giant WiFi umbrella around our world.

Today we have 24/7 connection to technology. I remember back before the advent of cell phones, when people left their houses, you simply couldn't get in touch with them until they returned home. If people were out, they would just stop by your house. "Hey! I was in the neighborhood and thought I'd stop by!" We were happy to have friends and family drop in for company.

Today, practically everyone in the developed world has a cell phone. It's attached to their hip most of the time, providing constant access to the infinite info of the Internet, and people around the world have nonstop access to you. Because of this increase in constant access, we've seen a correlating decrease in intimate connection. Sure, you can message people from anywhere at any time, but if you ever hear an actual knock on your door, you're probably like, "Who the heck is that?!" If someone is at home with you, you'll ask, "Are you expecting somebody?" while simultaneously trying to peek and see who it is and not being able to hide your annoyance. "Don't they know it's 2:00 p.m. on a Tuesday? Are they really just going to knock on the door like that?"

This may seem funny, and maybe you've seen this before, but even Grandma knows that she'd better text you before she comes over. And don't just pop up and text, "Hey, I'm in the driveway!" That just doesn't cut it. You can have round-the-clock access to me, but just make sure you give plenty of advance notice before you actually come over.

Our reliance on cell phones and other technology has changed the way we relate to each other and changed the way that our cells relate to each other, too. And the effects on children are far worse.

Unfortunately, children and teens are at greatest risk, both for parotid gland tumors and brain tumors, because their thinner skull bones allow for greater penetration of cell phone radiation.

The radiation can deeply impact tissues all the way to their midbrain, where tumors are more fatal. Additionally, children's cells reproduce faster, so they're more susceptible to aggressive cell growth. The biggest issue today is that kids face longer lifetime exposure. Many adults can clearly remember a time when cell phones didn't exist, whereas all the younger people alive today were born into the widespread use of cell phones. According to Lennart Hardell, MD, PhD, professor in the department of oncology at University Hospital in Örebro, Sweden, people who begin using cell phones heavily as teenagers have four to five times more brain cancer as young adults.

ELECTRONIC TEDDY BEAR

The moral of the story here: Don't keep cell phones around your body needlessly, and communicate this to the young people in your life as well. And, knowing these effects, why in the world would you sleep with your cell phone near you all night long?

People hang on to their phones and electronic devices like they are their best friends in the world. They act like they're going to fall over and die if they don't have their cell phones within texting distance.

Trust me, you'll live—and if you don't pay attention to this, all the rest of your years are not going to be very fun. Get the electronics *out* of your bedroom! If sleep is important to you, then you'll do this. If being healthy and not having a chronic disease is important to you, then you'll do this. Television, laptops, cell phones—all of these things are kicking out radiation that is disrupting your sleep. Have your entertainment in the entertainment area of your home. Keep your bedroom reserved for sleep and sex.

Numerous studies have confirmed that watching television before bed disrupts your sleep cycle. It might seem like a mundane activity to sit back and watch TV in your bed, but parts of your brain are being set off like fireworks. You're actually putting a stressor on your brain and body, especially if it's time to be winding down for bed.

Data show that children with televisions in their bedrooms score lower on school exams and are more likely to have sleep problems. And, to top it all off, having a TV in the bedroom is associated with a greater risk of obesity.

What about for mama and papa? Well, a recent study that tracked the sex lives of 523 Italian couples found that couples who don't have a TV in their bedroom have about twice as much sex as couples who do (this is the part of the book where some people smack themselves and then go and get the television out of their bedroom).

On the other side, people with TVs in the bedroom are generally having 50 percent less sex, and according to the research, after the age of 50, the decline is even more noticeable when a TV is present.

More and better sex should be reason enough for most people. I'll bet that after the world discovers this proven data, you'll be shocked if you see a television in a bedroom from then on. You'll walk into someone's bedroom, see a TV, then put your hand over your chest as you gasp and say, "Really? People still watch TV in bed . . . ? Really?"

And speaking of sex and electronics, a study published in the journal *Fertility and Sterility* found that 4 hours of wireless Internet-connected laptop exposure led to a significant decrease in progressive sperm motility and an increase in sperm DNA fragmentation. Sexual health and advanced technology don't mix very well (unless, of course, you're a robot from the future, and in that case, keep doing what you're doing!). It's these small things that we take for granted every day that can have a big impact on the results that we get.

Having these electronics in your bedroom is like a first-degree assault on your sleep and your body. Take action on this now, out of respect for your body, and get those gadgets out of your bedroom. Stack the conditions in your favor to ensure that you're creating an environment to get the sleep you deserve.

◇ ◇ ◇ ◇

FRIENDS OUT
POWER TIP #1

Many people use their phones as a Swiss Army knife to replace a lot of other useful devices. One of those useful devices is an alarm clock. To avoid this seduction of keeping your cell phone near your bedside, simply take action to use an actual alarm clock. You can use an alarm clock like I recommended in Chapter 10, with the full shut-off dimmer; you can use a traditional buzzer alarm clock; or you can even use a rooster for all I care. Just stop using your cell phone if you don't have to.

POWER TIP #2

Reminders about the importance of communication in a relationship have become cliché. Yet the reality of the situation is that communication is the basis for any successful union. If you want to get the TV out of your bedroom but you are worried that your partner won't want to go along with it, simply have a compassionate heart-to-heart with them. Explain why this is important to you, and ask them if they'd be willing to work with you on this because you respect them and want them to be happy as well. You'll probably be surprised what a little extra love and communication can do (plus, give them a copy of this book as a backup).

POWER TIP #3

It's suggested that things like televisions, stereos, air conditioner units, computers, and refrigerators be at least 6 feet away from your bed at night (that means 6 feet in the vertical sense, too!). If you're at all able to position your bed in a way that it achieves this recommended distance, then that's great. Sometimes there are extenuating circumstances, but always do the best you can with what you have right now.

Another potential issue can be the mattress itself. Research published in *Scientific American* states that, "In the United States, bed frames and box springs are made of metal, and the length of a bed is exactly half the wavelength of FM and TV transmissions that have been broadcasting since the late 1940s. Radiation envelops our bodies so that the maximum strength of the field develops 75 centimeters above the mattress in the middle of our bodies. When sleeping on the right side, the body's left side will thereby be exposed to field strength about twice as strong as what the right side absorbs."

Our mattresses can literally be a conductor of EMFs. That's not great news, but don't freak out. We'll talk a little bit more about mattresses in

Chapter 15, but if you already love the bed you're in, you can simply get some EMF shielding bed lining for use on your already existing mattress. This bed wear is shown to have a shielding effectiveness of 99.7 percent. You can find more information through the bonus resources at sleepsmarterbook.com/bonus.

FRIENDS OUT
POWER TIP #4

If you think there's a chance your sleep and your health are being affected by WiFi exposure in your home, simply get in the habit of turning off the WiFi at night. Biomechanist and bestselling author Katy Bowman utilizes a basic electrical timer to do this automatically. You simply install it in the socket where you plug your router in, and just set it to turn the power off during your preferred sleepy time. You can find more info about these easy-to-use electrical timers in the Sleep Smarter bonus resource guide as well.

FRIENDS OUT
POWER TIP #5

I know it might sound crazy, but everything will be okay if you keep your phone in another room while you sleep. It's 99.999 percent likely that you won't miss anything important. But, you *will* radically improve your sleep quality if you're not allowing your cell phone's notifications and radiation to disrupt your valuable sleep. Go on a cell phone free test drive. Just give it a shot for 1 week, and if the world ends while you're sleeping peacefully during that period, I'll try to call you the next day and let you know.

CHAPTER 13

LOSE WEIGHT AND DON'T FIND IT AGAIN

One of the most overlooked problems with getting great sleep is having too much body fat on your frame. Being overweight causes severe stress to your internal organs and nervous system, and it disrupts your endocrine system like few things can.

As we've discussed, your endocrine system (aka your body's hormonal system) is responsible for producing hormones like melatonin, oxytocin, and cortisol, which, as we've noted, have important roles in relation to sleep.

Let's take a look at the impact that being overweight has on cortisol, for example. Research presented by Deakin University in Australia showed that after consuming a meal, overweight individuals secreted radically higher levels of the stress hormone cortisol. People with a healthy weight showed a 5 percent increase in cortisol levels after consuming a meal, while overweight and obese individuals' cortisol levels increased by a whopping 51 percent! These high cortisol levels translate to higher blood sugar, lower insulin sensitivity, and increased levels of inflammation.

The biggest issue is that cortisol is as close to an anti-sleep hormone as you can get. Having higher levels of this stress hormone in your body will inherently damage normal function, no matter what time of day the meal is eaten. To know that each time you eat a meal your stress hormones are shooting through the roof is scary. This is one of the most important reasons to get the weight off, because it's killing you softly, like that old Fugees song.

The adage of not eating late at night if you want to lose weight actually has merit in this regard. But it's not that eating late at night is problematic in and of itself. It's when we are already overweight that it becomes a real concern. I should know—I've been on both sides of the spectrum.

EATING LATE AND BEING LEAN

I have a pair or two of fat genes. Pretty much everyone in my family while I was growing up was on the wrong side of 200 pounds, and this was horizontal weight, not vertical. For a time I got to see what my own fat genes looked like when I put them on. When I was dealing with the condition with my back, my body was puffy, painful, and seemingly paralyzed from lack of energy. It took so much to do so little. And when the tides changed, they changed in a big way.

I took my fat genes off and put some really nice genes on that I could get around in. I went from near 20 percent body fat to sub 7 percent body fat. It was crazy how effortless it seemed once I got momentum rolling, but the key was simply to get started in the first place!

While I was eating real food, being active every day, and sleeping like it was my long-lost love, I actually had a habit of eating late at night, every night. I'd eat a meal right around 10:00 p.m. before going to bed. The crazy thing was, I had never been so lean and healthy in my life. It's not that eating late is bad for weight loss, or that your body won't "burn it off," or any other popular idea like that. It's what's going on with your hormones that matters most, and when your hormones are in order, your life seems in order.

SO WHAT THE HECK ARE HORMONES ANYWAY?

Hormones are chemical messengers that deliver information throughout all the cells in your body.

Similar to what we talked about in Chapter 12, just one piece of data being off, just one small miscommunication, can lead to a totally different outcome. It's like that old game of telephone where one person starts with a message and whispers it into the ear of the next person, who continues to pass the message on. By the time it reaches the 10th person, the message could have gone from, "I can't wait to get some sleep tonight" to "I can't wait to date a sheep tonight."

Though counting sheep is synonymous with sleep, dating one is pretty weird, and not what the communication started out to be. In the same way, you might not intend for your body to do certain things, but when hormones are miscommunicating messages, things can get botched up really quickly.

The big secret that needs to be understood from this day forward is that you have a *huge* impact on what your hormones are doing every moment of your life.

Hormones are going to change their ratios and functions as you age. That's just a part of living. But what we've accepted as normal aging and normal health is anything but. We are either supporting normal hormone function or working against it with the decisions we make. We need to eat hormone-healthy foods, practice hormone-healthy exercise, and, as you now know, improve the quality of our sleep because it's one of the biggest navigators of our hormones overall.

My extra weight was definitely a contributor to my sleep problems. I knew this experientially, but the research shows it, too. Scientists at Johns Hopkins University School of Medicine conducted a study on people with reported sleep problems (such as sleep apnea, daytime fatigue, insomnia, and restless or interrupted sleep). Half of the volunteers went on a weight-loss diet with supervised exercise training. The other half did just the diet. After 6 months, participants in *both* groups had lost an average of 15 pounds and reduced their belly fat by 15 percent. As a result, the researchers found that each group equally boosted their sleep quality by about 20 percent, with a reduction in belly fat being the best indicator of improved sleep. This study also demonstrates that even without the vast benefits of exercise, the power of simply changing your diet has a huge impact on the results that you get.

THE DARK NIGHT

One of the more obvious issues that being overweight can have on sleep quality is *sleep apnea*. This is a sleep disorder characterized by pauses in breathing or infrequent breathing during sleep. Each pause in breathing, called an *apnea*, can last from at least 10 seconds to several minutes, and can occur from 5 to 30 times or more an hour. Basically, you stop breathing, and that results in abnormal blood pressure, depressed brain function, and dozens of other problems.

Neuroscientist and sleep disorder researcher Margaret Moline, PhD, states, "As the person gains weight, especially in the trunk and neck area, the risk of sleep-disordered breathing increases due to compromised respiratory function." Currently, more than 18 million Americans have sleep apnea, and several million more have severe organ stress and breathing problems due to the excess weight they're carrying around.

One of the common treatments for sleep apnea is to hook yourself to an assisted breathing machine known as a CPAP when you get into bed. These devices can be absolutely life-changing for some people in the short term, but with the increase in sleep quality and energy they provide, these machines should be a catalyst for addressing the real problem. Plus, some of the CPAP units basically make you look like Bane from *The Dark Knight Rises*. Cool if you're into that look, but it will likely have a negative impact on your love life.

The real solution is to not treat the symptom, but to address the underlying *cause* of most sleep apnea in the first place. Getting the excess weight off your frame is the key! When we talk about weight loss, we're talking about an issue that plagues millions of people worldwide each year. Good people, smart people, truly determined people, it doesn't matter. If you give a determined person the wrong map, they will inherently end up at the wrong destination.

That's what I've found to be the biggest problem when it comes to weight loss. There's a serious lack of honest, safe, and effective information. You have to understand that the weight-loss industry is a multibillion dollar industry, and it doesn't work well if there aren't lots of people struggling to figure this stuff out.

By using the backwards methods taught by many health gurus, the majority of people lose the weight and then they proceed to find it again. They work so hard to get the results they want, then eventually put the weight back on, and oftentimes a little bit more than they started with. If this is your story, then it's time now to step up and stop letting this happen to you.

I'm about to make this so easy that chances are you'll take it for granted. I've helped people lose thousands of pounds collectively *and* keep them off long term. What I'm going to share with you works. But you've got to make the decision to implement it.

THE LOWDOWN

If you're focusing on cutting calories to lose weight, then you might as well go and buy yourself some larger-size clothes right now. Research shows that up to 70 percent of the weight you lose through traditional calorie restriction is coming from a loss of your lean muscle tissue. As mentioned in Chapter 11, your muscle is your body's fat-burning machinery, and if you lose it through dieting, you'll depress your metabolism and set yourself up for long-term weight gain.

The problem is that people are thinking in terms of weight loss instead of *body-fat loss*. You don't want to lose weight. You want to lose fat. Remember, when it comes to this, *it's all about the hormones.*

You have to incite your body to secrete hormones that use stored body fat for fuel, and it's really as simple as that.

So how do we make this happen?

The first thing to understand is that you are either burning fat or storing fat—there is no in between. (Sounds very Zen, doesn't it?) If you're activating hormones that store fat all the time, then you're automatically throwing yourself out of the game, even if you're carefully counting your calories.

Your body's major fat-storing hormone is insulin. You may think of it only in regards to diabetes, but it's one of the most important hormones to your survival (and it can make you very fat if you don't know how to turn it off).

Now comes the easy part. The number one thing that insulin reacts to is carbohydrates. This includes all starches like bread, pasta, and potatoes; refined sugar products like cakes, candy, and soda; and even healthier carbohydrates like fresh fruit. To your body, it doesn't matter. These carbs come in, and insulin is turning on. Of course, an orange is better than orange sherbet in that it's delivering healthy vitamins and minerals as well, but the carb content is going to end up as glucose in the blood regardless.

To shift your body into more of a fat-burning state, you need to put more of your focus on the other two macronutrient groups: protein and fat. A study published in the *Journal of Nutrition* showed that increasing protein intake led to enhanced weight loss and improved blood fat levels. And a study in the *New England Journal of Medicine* split 132 people (many of whom had metabolic syndrome or type 2 diabetes) into either a low-carb group or a low-fat group for 6 months. The low-carb group lost an average of 12.8 pounds, while the low-fat group lost only 4.2 pounds. The lower-carb, higher dietary fat group literally lost three times as much weight!

It's not about having a low-carb diet necessarily; it's about having a better ratio of all three macronutrient groups for you and your unique metabolism. This seems pretty simple, right? So why aren't people doing this?

I was there on the front lines. I was sitting in the nutrition classes in college and being told *repeatedly* by my professors that we need to eat less fat and more carbohydrates to be healthy and maintain a healthy weight. You heard that right. They told me to have my clients do the exact *opposite* thing of what actually works. Side note: My professors were overweight, as were many of the other health professionals I worked with. Again, these are generally great people; they are smart people who were themselves taught the wrong thing. And if you teach a smart person how to do the wrong thing, they can become world class at doing the wrong thing. The education of health and nutrition in our world today is a whole other issue unto itself. The political reasons of why they were promoting a diet like that are not as important as you getting this information and using it to your advantage right now.

Dietary fats are critical to the normal function of your brain, nervous system, and endocrine system. It's just that fats have gotten a bad name because of, well, the name. People have grown to think that by eating fat, it ends up as fat on your body. This is sort of like thinking if you eat a bunch of blueberries, you will, in fact, turn blue. No disrespect to Smurfs, but it simply doesn't work like that.

A better word for dietary fats would be *energy*. The largest amount of structural fats is found in your nerve membranes, especially in the brain itself. Your brain is fat, and it's strutting its stuff! Fats are like insulation that wraps around nerve fibers, including the myelin that wraps around the fast-conducting nerve fibers in your brain that basically enable you to do everything that you do, but faster. Proteins, carbohydrates, and *energy* would lead to a much better marketing campaign to promote how important healthy fats are.

As far as weight loss, by eating a higher ratio of protein and healthy fats, you'll enable your pancreas to produce more *glucagon* instead of insulin.

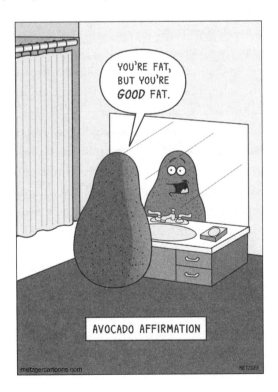

Glucagon triggers the breakdown of stored fatty acids for fuel and is essential to utilize if fat loss is your goal.

I want to keep this discussion focused on the topic of sleep as much as possible, so I'm not going to get into too much more detail here. If you've had a history of weight problems, or you simply want to be the leanest, healthiest version of yourself possible, then I highly recommend you head over and check out my program, The Fat Loss Code, at TheFatLossCode .com. It's an in-depth, 6-week training program complete with nutrition and exercise strategies that can be catered to you and your individual needs.

We are all unique, and understanding this is one of the most critical components of what works and what doesn't for weight loss. At the same time, there are still some consistent things to pay attention to across the board, because if you are human, then they are essential to you.

THE MICRONUTRIENT SECRET

There is so much talk today about the *macronutrients* we need to be in great shape that the amazing *micronutrients* are often overlooked. Micronutrients are things like the vitamins, minerals, trace minerals, phytonutrients, and enzymes that enable our bodies to function at their highest level. Simple micronutrient deficiencies like low magnesium can lead to overeating regardless of your macronutrient focus.

Also, micronutrients are essential to healthy hormone function, and remember, fat loss is all about the hormones! Eating micronutrient-rich foods can trigger your body to secrete more leptin (the satiety hormone) to keep you balanced, healthy, and in control. This is the exact opposite of most diets that restrict calories and advocate the use of micronutrient-deficient diet products like instant shakes, bars, and reduced-calorie pre-packaged snacks.

It doesn't matter that your pack of "healthy" processed cookies has only 200 calories. What is the quality of those calories, and what are they doing to your hormones? I'll tell you. They're basically kicking your hormones in the groin.

How do you get all of these micronutrient-rich foods?

Easy: By simply eating real food!

I told you I was going to make this easy, right? But how can you know if something is a real food or not? Well, I've put together a special little list for you.

Here's a simple list of things to help you know if it's a real food or not:

- If you can't tell where it comes from, chances are it's not real food (i.e., a bagel doesn't have any resemblance to a strand of wheat).
- If it comes through a drive-thru window, chances are it's not real food.
- If there are more than four or five ingredients, chances are it's not real food.
- If it even has to list the ingredients on it, chances are it's not real food.
- If it has a mascot or you get a special toy for buying it, chances are it's not real food.

Bottom line: To get the body you want to have, you have to get reconnected to nature. Your genes literally expect you to eat certain things. Once you get yourself reprogrammed through real food and smart exercise, there's literally no limit to how good things can get.

I KNOW YOU ARE, BUT WHAT AM I?

Being overweight or obese is a double-edged sword. Not only does obesity contribute to sleep problems, but sleep problems can also contribute to obesity.

A study out of Stanford University showed that when individuals were sleep deprived, they ended up with significantly decreased levels of leptin in their systems. Again, leptin is known as the satiety hormone because it plays such an important role in regulating appetite. Chances are, when you're tired or sleep deprived, this is the hardest time to resist the junk food that you know you should be avoiding.

When you're physically and mentally tired, your brain is looking for extra calories to keep everything functioning at a baseline level. Your brain knows that it can find those calories quickly and easily in chips, cookies, ice cream, and other kiddie foods that your grown-up butt suddenly can't resist. It's not an issue of willpower anymore; it's an issue of *survival* because the story goes deeper than this. . . .

Researchers discovered that sleep deprivation reduced the "higher order" functions of the brain and created excessive response in the primitive parts of the brain. Brain imaging scans done at University of California, Berkeley, showed that sleep deprivation caused more brain activity in the amygdala, an area associated with motivation to eat. The amygdala is very much a more emotional, reactive, survival-based part of the brain. This is how you can end up being *tungry* (tired and hungry). The study participants that these scans were taken from did, in fact, make poorer food choices.

Tie this together with reduced activity in the frontal cortex and insular cortex, the parts of the brain associated with evaluation, self-control, and rational decision-making. With these two changes in your brain due to sleep deprivation, you have a surefire recipe for struggle and failure.

You see, it isn't always about our willpower. So many really amazing and strong people fail at weight loss because they've unknowingly stacked conditions against themselves. When you're sleep deprived, your inner

SLEEP-DEPRIVED BRAIN WITH HIGHER ACTIVITY IN THE AMYGDALA

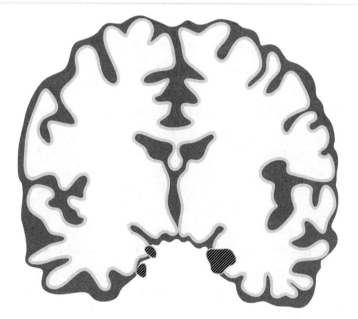

Incredible Hulk hijacks your brain, and you can't resist doing the very activity that you promised yourself you wouldn't do. You're tungry, and no one better stand in your way unless they want to get eaten, too.

Are your past diet failures your fault? Well, it really isn't a failure until you make an excuse. And it doesn't really matter if it was your fault if you were unaware. But, now that you know these critical insights to changing your body, you have to consciously stack the conditions in your favor to make future failures impossible.

Eve Van Cauter, PhD, professor of medicine at the University of Chicago, calls sleep deprivation "the royal route to obesity." Now understanding the fact that sleep deprivation decreases your insulin sensitivity, disrupts your hormonal cycles, and depresses your brain function, we know that her statement is 100 percent true. It's time to put all the excuses aside and give your body the sleep it requires to finally lose the weight and get the body and health you truly deserve.

SLEEP-DEPRIVED BRAIN WITH LESS ACTIVITY IN THE FRONTAL AND INSULAR CORTEX

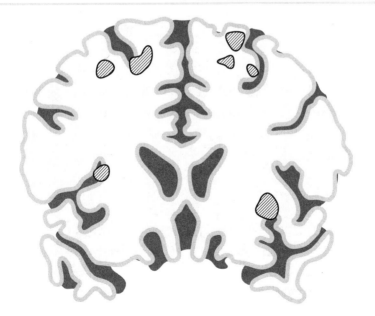

◇◇◇◇

LOSE WEIGHT WHILE SLEEPING
POWER TIP #1

If you really need to have something to eat closer to bedtime, have a high-fat, low-carb snack. This will ensure that your blood sugar stays stable. In contrast, if you eat a higher-carb snack right before bed, your blood sugar will spike, and the impending blood sugar crash can be enough to wake you up out of sleep. This is why, in our culture, we have the concept of waking up to get a "midnight snack." But hey, that's why they put a light in the refrigerator in the first place, right?

If you want to get truly restful sleep, one of the diciest things you can do is eat right before bed (especially if you're overweight, because cortisol levels go much higher). Give your body a solid 90 minutes (more is better) before heading off to bed after eating. Again, this is especially true if you're eating carbs, because if you're asleep when hypoglycemia hits, it will likely pull you out of deeper stages of sleep and make it difficult to drift back into them.

Again, it's not that carbs are inherently bad; it's just the timing of these things that can make all the difference. According to a study in the *American Journal of Clinical Nutrition*, eating easily digested carbs 4 hours before bedtime led people to fall asleep faster. After a good day of work, exercise, and time with family and friends, eating some of your favorite carbs along with a micronutrient-dense dinner could be a good thing. Just make sure that it's done a little earlier to give your blood sugar a chance to balance out.

LOSE WEIGHT WHILE SLEEPING
POWER TIP #2

Remember this always: Nutrient deficiency will lead to persistent overeating (which will lead to poor sleep and poor overall health).

In our society today it can be quite shocking how so many people are overwhelmed with calories, but starving for nutrition. When you find that you are continuously overeating, it's probably your body's cry for more nourishment. Your brain, organs, and cells are all driven by one thing: *survival*. Your brain and organs are constantly sharing data about specific nutrients that they need to function and regenerate themselves. Your body's hunger signals are controlled by your hypothalamus, which will simply send a shout-out to get those nutrients in. "Hey, we need potassium, B$_{12}$, copper, magnesium, and silica, stat!" Then, in comes a doughnut and coffee. Micronutrient increase reads: -82.

Not only did you not get the things your body needed, it actually lost more resources trying to process the fake food that came in! You got a few antioxidants from the coffee, but not enough to compare to the free radical activity caused by the doughnut.

So what does your body do in its infinite intelligence? It sounds the hunger alarm again. This time we need everything as before, but also calcium, selenium, lycopene, and vitamin C. In comes a sandwich and chips, and the whole thing keeps going on again and again. The person is constantly hungry, eating more and more food, and can't seem to find the off button. This is where the power of sleeping smarter and real food comes in to change the game.

By improving your sleep quality, you will inherently get an uptick in leptin sensitivity. And focusing on eating micronutrient-rich food as the bulk of your diet (with some room for fun stuff) will ensure that your body is producing leptin and filling the nutritional gaps that had you ravenously hungry in the first place. Game, set, match. You win.

LOSE WEIGHT WHILE SLEEPING
POWER TIP #3

Have your first meal be an epic one. Start your day off smart. Most people in our modern world have been programmed to start their day by having dessert for breakfast: oatmeal, toast, pancakes, bagels, cereal, fruit smoothies, and more. You're starting your day with a huge insulin spike and setting yourself up for a day of fat storage because of this.

Here we have one of the biggest secrets to long-term fat loss: *Keep insulin down through the first part of your day.* The morning is the ideal time to get in your real food, superfoods, and healthy fat supplements because you're right next to your cabinets at home. A breakfast of a vegetable omelet, sliced avocado topped with kelp granules (a sea veggie that's great for thyroid function), and some omega-3 supplements is a hormone-healthy way to start your day.

I'm not villainizing all smoothies, by the way, but if fat loss is your goal, you want to keep the fruit to a minimum (even though it's better than glazed doughnuts, it's still going to spike insulin if you're not careful about it). Instead, if you're going to make a smoothie, then make a green smoothie with a focus on the *green*. Load that blender up with a ridiculous amount of green leafy vegetables like spinach, some berries, protein powder, almond butter, some cacao powder (real chocolate powder), cinnamon, unsweetened almond milk, and maybe half a small banana or stevia to make it taste nice. The greens and micronutrients will help to keep that insulin response to a minimum.

Even though green smoothies are okay, the best breakfast option for most people is to go with some protein (like eggs, steak, or salmon), veggies (cooked and/or raw), and some healthy fats (like avocado, coconut, olives, or nuts and seeds). Stop having breakfast look like a meal served by Willy Wonka. If you want to lose fat, redefine your definition of a healthy breakfast, and start your body off in a fat-burning state, instead of a fat-storing state.

◇ ◇ ◇ ◇

Upgrading your nutrition, optimizing your hormone function, and preventing an amygdala hijack are all critical keys to improving your body and your sleep. But there is one important category of consumption that needs to be addressed to ensure that you get the best sleep possible. Let's jump right into the next chapter to find out what it is.

CHAPTER 14

GO EASY ON THE BOTTLE

Did you know that you actually get smarter while you sleep? One of the most valuable, but overlooked, aspects of sleep is a function called memory processing. This is where short-term memories and experiences get converted into long-term memories.

Memory processing is predominantly affected by different stages of REM sleep. If you get optimal REM sleep, all is well, but if your REM sleep is disrupted, your memory and your health can suffer.

Studies have proven the good news about drinking alcohol late in the evening is that you do, indeed, fall asleep faster. But the bad news is that REM sleep is significantly disrupted by alcohol being in your system. You won't be able to fall into deeper, consistent levels of REM sleep, and your brain and body won't be able to fully rejuvenate. This is why people generally don't feel that great after waking up from an alcohol-laced sleep.

You already know this to be true—that's why the word *hangover* has become so popular in our vocabulary today. And, of course, you've seen the movie *The Hangover*, right? That's just an extreme case of waking up not knowing what happened the night before (because you screwed up your memory processing), and possibly having a new tattoo on your face.

Research from the University of Missouri found that alcohol disrupts sleep by throwing off the body's balance of fatigue and wakefulness, something known as *sleep homeostasis.*

Homeostasis is essentially the ability to maintain internal stability. As you've seen, lack of sleep creates a "sleep debt" that's not so easily paid off. The best form of coin your body is shelling out to get you to go to sleep is adenosine, which we talked about in Chapter 4. As we discussed in that chapter, adenosine levels rise to encourage your body to go to sleep, but caffeine has the ability to block that sleepiness from happening. The result: You're sleepy but don't fully know it because caffeine has masked those feelings.

Adenosine is also a key player in the behavioral effects of alcohol, specifically in the promotion of sleep and the impairment of motor movements. Studies show that altered signaling of adenosine in the brain is involved in the pathophysiology of both alcohol dependence *and* sleep dis-

HEALTHY VERSUS ALCOHOL-RELATED SLEEP PATTERNS

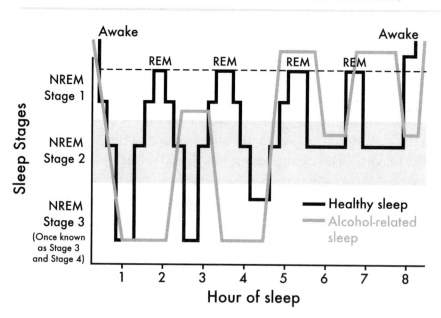

orders. Alcohol leads to increased extracellular concentrations of adenosine. The result: You're sleepy and you know it (and depending on how much alcohol you've had, you're sexy and you know it, too).

This artificial enhancement of adenosine throws off your sleep homeostasis as your body makes a concentrated effort to clean it all up. As you can see from the chart, alcohol consumption close to bedtime keeps sleep far below normal REM sleep during the first stage of sleep, and then there is a "REM rebound effect" that puts sleep above normal REM as your body is trying to sort things out. This is likely going to lead to you waking up feeling like a sock. An old, smelly, funny-colored tube sock. Sure, you went to sleep, but there's a big difference between getting high-quality sleep and passing out.

Now stretch this behavior out consistently, and we can see some real issues. Researchers at Washington University in St. Louis found that participants who had disrupted sleep cycles were more likely to show signs related to Alzheimer's disease than normal sleepers. This is another blatant cry to not mistake sleep quantity for sleep quality, and to avoid things that hurt your sleep and hurt your brain.

LADIES' NIGHT

There's strong evidence that drinking late in the evening is even more problematic for women. A study published in the journal *Alcoholism: Clinical and Experimental Research* had people drink alcohol in the name of science. Drinks were passed around to men and women, based on their weight, and everyone was equally drunk (measured by breath alcohol content). The findings showed that compared to the men, female participants woke up more often during the night, stayed awake longer, and slept for less time overall. This could be significant news if you're planning on doing shots for the next ladies' night out.

It's possible that alcohol affects women's sleep more because women metabolize alcohol faster than men do. Essentially, women can speed through alcohol's sedative effects quicker. If the alcohol is consumed close to bedtime, women can fall asleep faster, but the proceeding stages of sleep will have a much greater chance of being interrupted. In some cases, this can cause sweating, anxiety, or even nightmares (if they do happen to get any REM sleep).

Now, this isn't a get-out-of-jail-free pass for the fellas, nor is this an anti-fun stamp for the ladies. Drinking late at night affects everyone in some way; it's just about being able to navigate this fact to get the sleep we really need.

I GOTTA GO

One of the more obvious sleep interruptions from drinking alcohol before bedtime is the uncanny need to urinate. Getting up to relieve your bladder interrupts your sleep pattern because, well, you're peeing.

Every time you wake up from an alcohol-influenced sleep, it can be more difficult to fall back into the optimal sleep stages you need to recover. Bottom line: If you do drink closer to bedtime, be sure to give yourself ample time to go to the bathroom before turning in.

Drinking close to bedtime can also exacerbate current health problems you might be experiencing. Obviously, prostate and bladder problems come to mind, but what about diagnosed sleeping problems?

People with sleep apnea need to be careful here. Sleep disorder specialist Reena Mehra, MD, associate professor of medicine at the Cleveland Clinic Lerner College of Medicine of Case Western Reserve University, says that alcohol decreases muscle tone in the upper airway, meaning that breathing-related sleep issues are intensified after you've had a couple of drinks. People dealing with sleep apnea will tend to stop breathing more frequently and for longer periods of time after drinking. You have to consider if it's worth it because your chances of potential life-threatening side effects radically increase if you mix a cocktail of booze and sleep apnea.

As we discussed in Chapter 13, the real solution is to get the excess weight off of your frame to reverse the sleep apnea and improve your sleep quality. Drinking alcohol is synonymous with belly fat, so obviously this will not help in your weight-loss campaign. Am I saying not to go out and have fun with your friends? Of course not! But you have to get your priorities in order and take care of the things that are most important so that you can enjoy your time with your friends and family even more.

TIRED IS THE NEW VODKA

Another way that alcohol and sleep deprivation are intimately related is out on the road. Lisa Shives, MD, founder of Northshore Sleep Medicine in Evanston, Illinois, states, "Numerous studies have shown that sleepiness can impair driving skills as much as being drunk. In fact, being awake for 20 hours straight makes the average driver perform as poorly as someone with a blood alcohol level of 0.08 percent, now the legal limit in all states."

You know what it's like when the symptoms of drowsiness hit. Your head's nodding back and forth; you're losing awareness of things around you; your eyelids are becoming so heavy that it's a struggle to keep them open. Now, put a 4,000-pound driving machine at moderate to high speeds under your control. Yeah, it doesn't sound good. Because it's not.

The National Highway Traffic Safety Administration estimates that 100,000 crashes that are reported to the police each year are the direct result of fatigue and sleepiness. And this is actually a conservative number because testing for drowsiness isn't remotely as easy as testing blood alcohol levels.

Drunk driving is an international concern that's impacted the lives of far too many people. Because of it, awareness has grown, and substantial measures have been taken to help prevent it. But who is advocating against people driving with extreme fatigue? A recent National Sleep Foundation poll found that 60 percent of drivers admitted that they had driven while sleepy in the preceding year, and 37 percent confessed that they had fallen asleep behind the wheel. What could be more dangerous than that?! Data shows that many accidents involving fatigued drivers who've fallen asleep don't show skid marks in an effort to avoid the accident, and a large number of these types of accidents are hard to track because they are often fatal.

Another recent study conducted by the AAA Foundation for Traffic Safety uncovered that drowsy drivers are responsible for one in six—or 17 percent—of fatal car accidents. But because being sleep deprived and driving is something that's culturally accepted, while being drunk and driving is something that is frowned upon, this type of surprising data can still seem a bit far-fetched. Well, the kings of cracking far-fetched set out to see if driving while tired is really that dangerous. The Discovery Channel's

MythBusters took to the case to see how driving intoxicated and driving tired really compared.

For the project, MythBusters Tory Belleci and Kari Byron got a baseline test of performance on two different courses. One simulated city driving conditions, and one was a more monotonous course to simulate highway driving (involving 25 laps around a track) to evaluate the drivers' attention spans.

The test was monitored by a police officer on a closed course, and the MythBusters confessed that it was likely the most dangerous experiment they've done. Tory and Kari consumed enough alcohol to put them just under the legal limit at almost 0.07 percent and then hit the two courses while "tipsy" to set a baseline in performance. After the baseline was set, the next part of the experiment required the two to stay up for 30 straight hours. So they stayed up right through the night and then retook the test. The results were absolutely shocking.

Compared with driving around while tipsy, sleep deprivation caused Tory to drive *10 times* worse, while Kari's driving was *3 times* more erratic (her baseline while driving tipsy wasn't good to begin with, but driving while sleep deprived hit her even harder). Though this example is moving to more serious levels of sleep deprivation, how often are people driving with at least some level of significant fatigue that's impairing their ability to operate the multiple-ton vehicle under their body?

This is a PSA to let you know that it's just not worth it. And also to think about what else people are doing while sleep deprived. Building roads and bridges, performing surgeries, inspecting our food and water supply, driving buses and taxis . . . the list goes on and on. When we are not caring for ourselves and putting a priority on sleep, we can become more of a danger to ourselves *and* the people around us.

This chapter is important because it's a reality check. We take things like driving and being able to consume alcohol for granted. We know that the two don't play nice together. But neither does alcohol and sleep—and neither does sleep deprivation and driving. This does not mean that you can't have an amazing time hanging out with friends and family, but you need to have a smart plan of action to make sure that you stay healthy at the end of the day.

◇ ◇ ◇ ◇

EASY ON THE BOTTLE
POWER TIP #1

Wrap up the drinks at least 3 hours before hitting the sack. If you want to play at a high level and still hang out with your friends for drinks, then hook up with them for happy hour instead of an all-night bender.

If you want to be a champ at this rejuvenating sleep thing, consider having a booze curfew so that your body can have a few hours to get it out of your system before you go to sleep. The amount you drink, your weight, and your body fat will play a role in exactly how long that is. There's a great alcohol metabolism rate chart and blood alcohol level calculator in the Sleep Smarter bonus resource guide at sleepsmarterbook.com/bonus.

EASY ON THE BOTTLE
POWER TIP #2

Practice sleeping smarter to get the rest and recovery your body really needs so that you don't put yourself in a dangerous driving position in the first place. Extenuating circumstances can happen, though, so if you have the symptoms of sleepiness coming on strong, just pull the car over. Board-certified sleep medicine physician Dr. Lisa Shives says, "Find a safe place and try to take a 10- to 20-minute nap. Studies have shown that shorter naps result in greater alertness and better performance." Experts also recommend avoiding driving alone for long distances late at night. And the National Sleep Foundation recommends taking a break every 2 hours if you are driving on a long road trip.

EASY ON THE BOTTLE
POWER TIP #3

Drink more . . . water, that is.

Alcohol is assimilated into your blood very quickly, in part because it's in liquid form. To help nullify the effects of the alcohol faster, you need to drink more water to help flush out the metabolic waste products left behind.

Alcohol is also a diuretic, meaning it will cause your body to expel more fluids and increase your likelihood of dehydration. For every alcoholic drink you have, your body can eliminate up to four times as much liquid. Dehydration is one of the primary causes of nausea and other nonappealing symptoms of a hangover.

To recover faster and keep your body hydrated, wine expert Anthony Giglio recommends having one 8-ounce glass of water with every alcoholic drink that you consume. Keeping a pitcher of water at your table doesn't take *Jeopardy*-level intelligence, but I bet you'll feel like a genius when you wake up the next day without a hangover.

CHAPTER 15

PLAY YOUR POSITION

I t might seem surprising to need to talk about sleeping positions. Most people think that it's as simple as laying their butt down and then the magic will happen from there. We tend to not think about the importance of our sleeping position because it's something that we've done for so long that it's become automatic.

The reality is that your sleeping position matters. A lot.

Here are just some of the things that are affected by your sleeping position:

- Bloodflow to your brain
- Stability of your spine
- Hormone production
- Joint and ligament integrity
- Oxygen supply and efficient breathing
- Muscular function and healing
- Heart function and blood pressure
- Digestion and cellular metabolism

If you're sleeping in a position that compromises your body's ability to function and recover, it doesn't matter how many hours of sleep you get,

THE MOST POPULAR SLEEPING POSITIONS

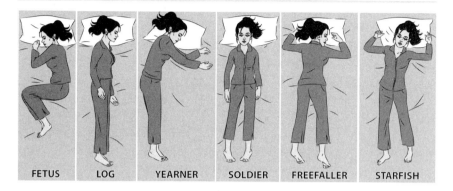

| FETUS | LOG | YEARNER | SOLDIER | FREEFALLER | STARFISH |

you're still going to feel like a piñata the day after the party when you wake up.

One of the most important facets of your sleeping position is maintaining the integrity of your spine. Any good chiropractor can educate you on the fact that the brain stem running through your spine is directly connected to every major organ in your body. If your spine is compromised and there's a break in the information between your brain and your body, chronic and catastrophic problems can take place. Some of these problems can be rooted in the way you're sleeping.

There are many flavors of sleeping positions that people use to get their beauty sleep. From the Starfish position, to the Free-Faller, to the Soldier, there are many ways to get cozy in bed.

Even though there are many sleeping styles that people put themselves in, there are only one or two that we tend to gravitate toward personally. Have a look at the chart and see which sleeping style you tend to use.

There are many variations of these positions, but these are the basics. And to make it even simpler, we're just going to focus on getting you in the best position on your back, your stomach, or your side.

HAVE YOUR OWN BACK

Many experts will tell you that sleeping on your back is the ideal position to be in. There are several reasons that this could be accurate. First of all, your spine can be in the best position here (as long as you don't make some of the mistakes we'll talk about in a moment). You will also have less likelihood of digestive distress, like acid reflux, in this position. And, for all those who are cosmetically conscious, sleeping on your back allows your facial skin to breathe, so you'll be less prone to having breakouts and early-onset wrinkling.

The downside of sleeping on your back is the greater likelihood of snoring and sleep apnea. This is partly because when we sleep on our backs, gravity can force the base of the tongue to collapse into the airway, obstructing normal breathing. Another reason for this is general throat weakness that's exacerbated by lying on your back, causing the throat to close during sleep. If someone has too much body fat on their frame (as we discussed in Chapter 13), fat gathering in and around the throat can cut off the normal air supply. Losing excess body fat and utilizing a different sleep position can help to remedy this.

Back-sleeping is the most politically correct choice, but, admittedly, not the most comfy position to be in. It's definitely safer for your spine, but it's not the best position if you're making either of the following big mistakes:

Using a huge pillow: Some people's beds look like a full-on pillow fiesta. It's okay to have a bunch of pillows for decoration, but this does *not* mean that you have to sleep on all of them. Having a pillow or pillows that are too big under your head while lying on your back totally misaligns the natural curve of your spine. You can end up with neck pain, back pain, headaches, or even worse. You'll also have poor circulation to your brain all night because the blood is trying to move uphill past Mount Pillow.

A natural position during sleep would mean having your head lower because this is the one time that your body shouldn't have to work harder to pump blood to your brain. Break the pillow addiction immediately because it's bad business for your back and your brain.

Using a worn-out mattress: Seriously, you're better off sleeping on the floor. The mattress is supposed to support you—not too much (like the floor) and not too little (like having your butt sink into a fluffy abyss). You don't have to get the most fancy-pants mattress in the world; just make sure that you're not sinking in so much that your spine's natural curve is compromised. We'll talk more about mattresses shortly.

SLEEP LIKE A BABY

Sleeping on our stomachs used to be synonymous with sleeping like a baby. Laying infants on their stomachs to sleep has gone in and out of favor and is still much debated in our world today. Child development specialist Dr. Václav Vojta states that lying on our stomach as infants is actually critical to our development. Through 50 years of research, Dr. Vojta identified that there are specific pressure points on our bodies that "activate" nervous system programs when we are infants. These pressure points are engaged when children are allowed to lie on their bellies and do subtle movements that they would naturally do while sleeping.

Update that to our adulthood, and many people just feel more comfortable and peaceful lying on their bellies. There are many pros and cons to this, so if you're going to do it, do it right.

Lying down face-first with your legs straight and your arms right by your sides is probably a bad idea. This is compromising your back by taking away the natural curve of your lumbar spine. Add having your head to one side, smashed into a pillow for hours on end, and you've got a serious recipe for disaster.

On the brighter side, some research shows that lying on your stomach can help prevent minor snoring and some symptoms of sleep apnea. Sleeping belly-down keeps your upper airways more open, so this could be okay for you if you follow a few simple rules:

Lift a knee: Lift one knee up to open your hips and take some of the pressure off your spine from lying with your legs straight.

Lose the pillow: If you're going to sleep on your belly, then ditch the pillow, because you really don't need it. Using a pillow will hyperextend your neck all night, and that's just silly. Think of walking around all day with your head tilted back looking at the sky. Yes, you'll look crazy, but you'll also have neck problems.

Use the pillow for something else: Placing a small, firm pillow underneath your belly and hips will reduce the stress on your low back and neck. Simply place a pillow in a comfortable spot on the same side that you've lifted your leg, and you're in a much healthier position to sleep on your stomach.

ON THE WINNING SIDE

Most people report that they prefer to sleep on their side, and for good reason. Our most intense times of sleep and development happened while we were in the womb, curled up in the fetal position. Sleeping on our side is the natural sleeping position to emulate this developmental template.

Side-sleeping can be a quick fix for snoring and can help to improve breathing, more so than lying on your back. Plus, sleeping on your side (the left side in particular) has been reported to ease troublesome digestive problems like acid reflux and heartburn.

The downside, as most side-sleepers know, is the dreaded "dead-arm" and finger numbness from this position. Sleeping on your arm for too long can cut off bloodflow and nerve function. You can wake up feeling that someone played a prank on you and slathered your arm with novocaine.

Here are some simple tips for sleeping on your side:

Shoulder lean: Instead of sleeping with your shoulder directly under you, move it forward slightly to avoid constriction of your shoulder and arm muscles.

Pillow proposition: Make sure that your head isn't propped up too high on pillows. You want to ensure that you're maintaining the natural straight position of your spine with a pillow that supports your neck, but doesn't raise your head too much.

For those with back pain: Experts recommend sleeping on your side with a soft pillow between your knees if you have a history of back problems. This helps to stabilize your spine and alleviate pressure from your hips and lower back.

HOT BED OF QUESTIONS

Approximately one-third of your entire life will be spent on the mattress you choose to sleep on.

The importance of this sleeping surface cannot be overstated. Now, just to be clear, even being able to choose your mattress is a great gift. Many people across the world sleep on the ground, yet sleep more peacefully than people on the highest-priced beds. We have to put things in perspective and

SPINAL ALIGNMENT BASED ON MATTRESS RESILIENCY

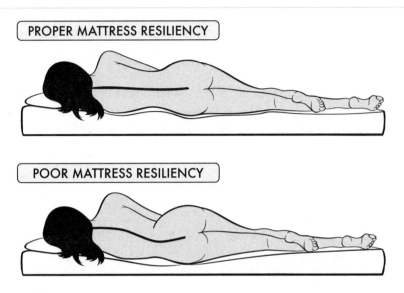

PROPER MATTRESS RESILIENCY

POOR MATTRESS RESILIENCY

know that the bed is important, yes, but the other things in this book matter just as much. That said, your mattress can either be a source of more problems, or a truly health-giving gift that makes the other two-thirds of your life even better.

Research indicates that more than 70 million Americans suffer from sleep-related pain. Instead of waking up feeling refreshed, millions of people are waking up with aches and pains due to the mattress they've been sleeping on. *Consumer Reports* states that you need to replace your mattress every 7 years, but this is something that most of us just don't take into account. We get a mattress, go on about our lives, and usually don't give it a second thought.

One of the biggest reasons that switching out your mattress every 7 years is recommended is that most mattresses sag 25 percent within the first 2 years, and they continue to degrade rapidly from there. This has been found to be the greatest contributor to sleep-related back pain.

When you're lying down, your hips are the heaviest part of your body, so mattresses layered with foam break down and degrade there first and lose what's known as their *mattress resiliency* (its ability to push back). Inconsistent push-back leads to problems with your spinal integrity and disorganized muscle tension within your hips and spine. You may think you're relaxed, but because of the uneven distribution of your weight, some muscles are relaxed, while other muscles are on *all night long*, as Lionel Richie might say.

At first the mattress will feel fine, but over time it loses its resiliency, and you might not even realize that problems you're having are related to where you lay your head down at night. It's not just back pain, but neck problems, issues with internal organs, and even your risk of injury during your waking hours all increase when your body gets out of sorts from a tired mattress. But even this might not be the biggest concern.

WINDOW DRESSING

Many people are shocked to find out that most mattresses contain toxic foams and synthetic fabrics, and are treated with chemical flame retardants that off-gas and lead to a whole host of health problems.

Chemicals in conventional mattress flame retardants include:

- **PBDEs (polybrominated diphenyl ethers):** Used in mattresses before 2004. However, since it was determined that these chemicals are toxic to your liver, thyroid, and nervous system, mattress companies have phased use out.
- **Boric acid:** Has known carcinogenic properties.
- **Melamine resin (contains formaldehyde):** The US Environmental Protection Agency (EPA) classified formaldehyde as a probable human carcinogen under conditions of prolonged exposure.

If you've ever had a mattress delivered, many times they'll tell you to "let the room air out" after setting it up. Call me a dreamer, but I don't think your bedroom should smell like it was freshly painted after getting a mattress delivered. We are also under the impression that once you can't smell it anymore, it's now perfectly safe, but this is simply not the case.

Something that started with good intentions (flame retardants) came with far more probable health concerns. The impact on adults is concerning, but the impact on children is far greater.

Renowned scientist and chemist James Sprott, PhD, believed that though crib death can result from a variety of causes, one of the biggest concerns are toxic gases that are generated from a baby's mattress. He asserted that chemical compounds containing phosphorus, arsenic, and antimony have been added to mattresses as fire retardants and for other purposes since the early 1950s. Funguses that commonly grow in bedding can interact with these chemicals to create poisonous gases. Once a baby breathes or absorbs a lethal dose of the gases, the central nervous system can shut down, stopping breathing and then heart function. These gases can fatally poison a baby, without waking the child and without any struggle. And, according to Dr. Sprott's research, a normal autopsy would not reveal typical signs that the baby was poisoned.

This is quite alarming, but it's a call to pay attention to detail and the things we've accepted as normal. One thing he mentioned was not just breathing in, but *absorbing* these materials. It's important to understand that if you can smell something, then it's on your skin and in your body. (That might freak you out the next time someone passes gas around you. I'm sorry, but it's true!) But we also become desensitized to smells very quickly. Our olfactory senses down-regulate our experience of smells rapidly whether they are good or not so good. This is why it's often said to stop and smell the roses, because you won't be able to notice them very long if you don't.

As mentioned, just because you can't smell something doesn't mean that it's safe. This is why it's of the utmost importance to start choosing mattresses that don't pose the risks that we've discussed. Mattresses are generally something we'll just pass along, like old shoes or clothes, but research published in the *British Medical Journal* has shown that the reuse of infant mattresses triples the risk of crib death. This is because whenever anyone sleeps on a mattress, skin cells are shed by the body that can become organic matter for microbes to decompose. What can result is a microbial, toxic dance-off that can silently pose a great risk to our health.

A really important nationwide program took place in New Zealand to protect children and prevent SIDS in 1994. Understanding the startling data regarding the hazards of off-gassing mattresses, health-care professionals throughout New Zealand actively advised parents to wrap their new baby's mattress in an inexpensive, nontoxic protective cover. Over the following 20-year span, there was not one single SIDS death reported among the more than 200,000 New Zealand babies who slept on mattresses wrapped with the protective cover. There were 1,020 crib deaths reported since the mattress-wrapping campaign began, but none of them were children whose beds were properly wrapped.

As you can see, your choice in a mattress for yourself or your loved ones isn't something to just glance over. Sure, your bed might have 37.7 layers of foam and a mystical pillow top that molds itself around you like a bodysuit, but that's just window dressing. How long does the resiliency of your mattress really last? And was your mattress treated with potentially toxic materials that you should be concerned about?

Make sleeping on a nontoxic mattress a priority. Make sleeping on a mattress that maintains its resiliency much longer a priority. A mattress is usually a big investment in our lives, so the next time you make the decision to purchase a mattress for yourself or your family, be sure to follow my recommendations in the Sleep Smarter bonus resource guide at sleepsmarterbook .com/bonus. They will be incredibly helpful for you.

In the meantime, utilizing mattress covers for babies and small children is a great idea. You can get more information on those through the bonus resource guide as well, so head over there and check it out. Sleep healthy, sleep safe, and sleep smarter!

ARE YOU SLEEPING WITH YOUR SOUL MATE, OR SLEEPING WITH THE ENEMY?

Oftentimes, sleeping with someone you love is a great comfort. There's nothing better than going to sleep with, and waking up with, your favorite person each day. But, take notice. If you want to keep them as your favorite person, and continue to be theirs, you have to navigate this sleep situation with intelligence.

Make no mistake: Sleeping in a bed with another live body can make for an entertaining experience. Some people can get along in the bed just fine, while other people prepare to go into battle each night. Some people are peaceful and don't move much; others act as though they're an acrobat in

Cirque du Soleil. Some people hog the covers, some people snore, some people talk in their sleep, some people even scream out loud. The relationship goes to a whole new level when you meet somebody's sleep alter ego.

Obviously, communicating and following the guidance in this book is going to be invaluable. But what about the sleeping position itself? Unless you have a double California king-size bed, the Starfish position isn't going to cut it.

To make this really easy, this chart will provide you with some sleep positions to try. Simply test them out and find which one(s) work best for you and your partner so that you can both get the best sleep possible.

THE MOST POPULAR COUPLES SLEEPING POSITIONS

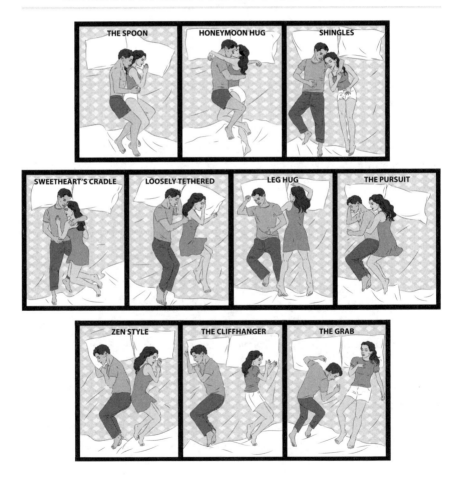

◇ ◇ ◇ ◇

POWER TIP #1

Our sleep position habits are just like any other habits: They can take some time to change. Start off the night in your ideal sleep position, and if you wake up during the night and find yourself in a position that you don't want to be in, simply make a conscious effort to get into one that you prefer.

POWER TIP #2

Make sure to communicate your sleeping needs and preferences to your partner—this simply cannot be emphasized enough. Talk to them with intention and compassion. Understand their sleeping needs, and make sure that you're doing what you can to make them feel comfortable, too.

There are few things more intimate in life than sharing a sleeping space with someone else. It can create a greater connection, or it can create more irritation than you can imagine. The simple solution is to communicate with love and respect.

POWER TIP #3

Set your sights on getting a nontoxic, non-off-gassing mattress that has a higher level of resiliency than the industry standard if at all possible. Again, you spend about one-third of your entire life on the mattress you choose, so make sure that it's one that's adding to your health and not taking away from it. Get the resource guide at sleepsmarterbook.com/bonus and use it to your advantage.

CHAPTER 16

CALM YOUR INNER CHATTER

There is a great quote that says, "My bed is a magical place where I suddenly remember everything I was supposed to do."

People hop into bed and then proceed to think about the when, where, who, why, what, and how of their life . . . all while they're supposed to be sleeping. If this sounds familiar to you, then you have a serious issue with something we call *inner chatter*. But don't worry, there is a solution.

It's important to realize that there is nothing "wrong" with you just because you have a lot of thoughts. It's part of being human. It's actually a great gift to be able to process as much information as we do. Experts estimate that we have upwards of 50,000 thoughts per day, most of them random, and most of them short-lived. But, in our overinformed, overstressed, and hyper-sensitized world today, it can all be a bit much. We need to learn to turn the volume down when we want to. And it's really as simple as that.

What I'm going to share with you is not just a tool to help you improve your sleep; it's a powerful tool to help transform your life overall. The inner chatter that you experience is a result of the stress and untamed busyness of the day. Now, more than ever, with the constant flow of information coming at you, it's important to have a practice to help you buffer that stress. That important practice is *meditation*.

TRAIN YOUR BRAIN

Meditation doesn't have to be complicated, and it definitely doesn't require that you subscribe to any weird beliefs; you don't have to sit cross-legged on the floor for hours, you don't have to quit shaving, you don't have to change your name to a symbol or a fruit, and you don't have to drink any Kool-Aid whatsoever.

Meditation or *brain training*, as I like to call it, can be as simple as sitting quietly and focusing on your breathing, or counting your steps as you walk around the park. You can even turn everyday activities like taking a shower or washing your clothes into a great meditation by following a few basic principles.

Meditation is like a tonic. A tonic is something that you can use every day, and the results continue to get better and better. The more you meditate, the more calm and presence you'll have in your day-to-day life.

Now when I say *more*, I'm talking about frequency, and not a specific time requirement. Once you find the right meditation for yourself, you can almost instantly feel a sense of calm and presence by doing your practice throughout the day.

I started off meditating for 30 to 45 minutes every morning for 3 years. Today, I do more "mini-meditations," often 5 minutes or less, and I feel the same focus and peace that I felt all those years when meditating for a half hour or more. How? Because the effects are cumulative, and the neuro-association my brain and body have made to closing my eyes and focusing on my breath instantly puts me in that relaxed space.

Numerous studies show that meditation increases "feel-good" hormones and endorphins, lowers stress hormones like cortisol, and even reduces inflammation in the body. Now, you can buy stuff that can give you similar experiences, but it'll probably cost you a lot of money (and you might get arrested for it, too).

Let's take a look at the proven ways that a meditation practice can improve your life.

Performance

In a study published in the journal *Brain Research Bulletin*, researchers discovered that people trained to meditate over an 8-week period were better able to control specific types of brain waves called alpha rhythms.

The lead author of the paper, MIT neuroscientist Christopher Moore, PhD, stated, "These activity patterns are thought to minimize distractions, to diminish the likelihood stimuli will grab your attention. Our data indicate that meditation training makes you better at focusing, in part by allowing you to better regulate how things that arise will impact you."

Could you use more focus in your life right now? Would being less distracted be helpful to you?

If you're like most people, then focus is a huge issue. Our ability to focus and get things done is a big component of overall success. Meditation literally changes your brain and enables you to utilize your ability to focus like nothing else can. Not in an "oh, that sounds nice" kind of way, but by actually changing the way your brain grows and operates.

After 8 weeks, compared to a control group, the subjects who had been trained in meditation showed larger changes in the size (amplitude) of their alpha waves when asked to focus on one specific thing. Essentially, their focus was stronger and deeper than at the beginning of the study. Researchers at Harvard Medical School have also found that meditation alters the structure of your brain, thickening the regions associated with attention and sensory processing.

There is an absurd amount of data mounting about the beneficial impact of meditation on work performance, productivity, memory, and focus. Don't be the one who misses the boat because you didn't take advantage of this valuable resource.

Health

Research at the Medical College of Georgia in Augusta found that meditation lowered blood pressure and reduced the risk of heart disease and stroke. Numerous studies also demonstrate that meditation can reduce chronic pain and associated inflammatory biomarkers.

Today, more than 80 percent of physician visits are for stress-related illnesses. Stress is at the top of the list of reasons why people begin a meditation practice. Countless studies show the stress-reducing effects in healthy individuals, as well as in patients suffering from a variety of diseases. Meditation has proven to be good for your brain, good for your body, and good for life overall.

Sleep

The American Academy of Sleep Medicine published research showing that meditation is an effective treatment for insomnia. The study showed that over a 2-month period, sleep latency, total sleep time, total wake time, wake after sleep onset, sleep efficiency, sleep quality, and depression improved in patients who used meditation.

The principal investigator in the study, Ramadevi Gourineni, MD, stated, "Results of the study show that teaching deep relaxation techniques during the daytime can help improve sleep at night."

Another study, published in the journal *Medical Science Monitor*, found that advanced meditators have higher baseline melatonin levels than nonmeditators.

The most important takeaway is that the only side effect associated with meditation is a better quality of life. In contrast, jumping right to drugs to treat insomnia is associated with organ damage, hormone disruption, and significant chemical dependency. Why deal with those potential downsides when there are better—and safer—actions that you can take first?

RIDE THE WAVE

We all have four different brain wave frequencies that are most often expressed, measured in cycles per second (Hz). Each of these brain wave frequencies has its own set of characteristics that demonstrate specific brain activity and a unique state of consciousness. Here is a brief description of the four:

Beta waves (15 to 40 Hz): This is the brain rhythm in the normal state of wakefulness, associated with thinking, conscious problem-solving, and attention toward the outer world. You are most likely in a "beta state" while reading this right now.

Alpha waves (9 to 14 Hz): When you are truly relaxed, your brain waves slow from the hyper-alertness of beta waves to the gentle waves of alpha. The "alpha state" is where meditation begins, and it's a brain wave frequency that heightens your imagination, visualization, memory, learning, and concentration. This is the gateway to the subconscious mind and reprogramming your thinking.

Theta waves (4 to 8 Hz): Theta brain waves are present during deep meditation and light sleep, including the important REM dream state. This is the domain of your subconscious and only experienced momentarily as you drift off to sleep from alpha *or* wake from deep sleep (delta waves). We are more receptive to insights and information beyond our normal conscious awareness in this state. Some experts state that theta meditation amplifies intuition and other extrasensory perception skills.

THE FOUR PRIMARY HUMAN BRAIN WAVE STATES

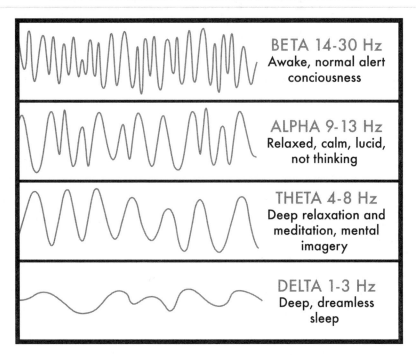

BETA 14-30 Hz
Awake, normal alert
conciousness

ALPHA 9-13 Hz
Relaxed, calm, lucid,
not thinking

THETA 4-8 Hz
Deep relaxation and
meditation, mental
imagery

DELTA 1-3 Hz
Deep, dreamless
sleep

Delta waves (1 to 3 Hz): The delta frequency is the slowest of the frequencies and is experienced in deep, dreamless sleep. It is also seen occasionally in very experienced meditators. The delta state is critical to the body's healing processes. Much of our regeneration and healing happen in this brainwave state, making getting enough deep sleep critical to our survival.

The ability to change your brain waves is one of the reasons meditation works. You can consciously, proactively change the way your brain operates, and the potential benefits are tremendous. Yet another important reason meditation works is the instant change to your autonomic nervous system.

BREATHING FOR THE WIN

Food is important. But you can go weeks without it. Water is important. But you can go days without it. We can only go a few *minutes* without oxygen. It's the most critical component to our health and survival. Breathing is how we get it in and process it, but most of us breathe like we're talking to someone with bad breath and don't want to fully take in the stink.

We tend to breathe shallow and short, barely giving our bodies the oxygen that it needs. But now that we've been talking about breathing, you've probably become more conscious of your breathing, haven't you? You've probably taken a deep breath or two. The crazy thing is . . . were you not breathing before? Of course you were! But it was running on autopilot.

Your breathing is part of your autonomic nervous system, which is a system that acts largely unconsciously. It regulates things like cardiac function (aka beating your heart), digestion, dilation and contraction of the pupils in your eyes, and, of course, respiration. I don't know about you, but I don't want the responsibility of consciously beating my heart and digesting my food. It would be an unearthly challenge if we had to do that. However, controlling your breath is something very different.

We have an autopilot that operates our breathing, but at any time we can jump in and grab the controls. We can make our breathing deeper, more shallow, faster, slower, and variations of it all. We can consciously control our breathing, but why? Evolutionarily speaking, it's to our advantage because our temporary perception doesn't always equal our reality.

BREATHE LIKE A BABY

The autonomic nervous system is regulated by your hypothalamus (again, that master gland that modulates stress) and is the primary mechanism in control of your fight-or-flight response. When fight-or-flight is activated, your muscles tense, your heart rate increases, your pupils dilate, bloodflow is constricted to many parts of your body, digestion in your stomach and upper intestinal tract slows down or stops altogether, and your breathing becomes faster and shorter.

This incredible fight-or-flight response is a physiological reaction that occurs in response to a perceived harmful event, attack, or threat to survival. It's a huge evolutionary advantage because it instantaneously shuts down bodily processes that are not critical to short-term survival, and heightens bodily processes that are. You now have the enhanced capability to fight that man-eating lion, or run for the hills to find cover. To put it simply, fight-or-flight is the polar opposite of relaxation and sleep.

The key words here are *perceived* harmful event, attack, or threat to survival. Your perception is your reality. Even if it's not true. Have you ever been walking outside and almost jumped out of your skin because you thought you saw a snake, but it was really just a stick? Your fight-or-flight system kicked into high gear, but there was no problem to begin with. Stress hormones shot up, but it was just a misinterpretation of your environment. This is a physical example, but the psychological examples are far more prominent.

Worry over a job interview, potential layoff, missing a flight, negative comments on social media, loss of money or an inability to pay a bill, the health and well-being of people you care about, traffic jams, work deadlines, and on and on and on . . . Even though these things hardly ever really hurt us, many of us worry about them on a daily basis. All of the things that stress us out and create fear are activating our fight-or-flight system. Just because we *perceive* them as a threat, the fight-or-flight system is turning on and our body is experiencing the effects.

Basically, today we don't have to worry about man-eating lions for the most part, so with that freed-up space we have a tendency to manufacture things to worry about. Again, it's not our fault if we're unaware. But once you know this stuff, it becomes your responsibility to change it.

We've evolved to hunt and look out for any potential danger to keep us safe. Now billions of us don't have to hunt and look for food. Our biggest danger is choosing what restaurant to eat at with a significant other who's incredibly indecisive. It's like that scene in the movie *The Notebook*. You: "What do you want?!" Them: "It's just not that simple!"

Now understanding how our primitive programming and old habits can hijack our brains, it's time to take back control.

The big thing to remember is that the *sympathetic* nervous system (the fight-or-flight system) is a binary system, meaning that it's either off or it's on. It can't be *sort of* on. It's either on or it's not (just at varying degrees). When it's off, the counter side of this system is the *parasympathetic* nervous system, appropriately known as the rest and digest system. Just as you can influence if the sympathetic system is turned on, you can activate the parasympathetic system, too. And the breath is the key.

We can literally put ourselves in a stress response with shallow breathing and not even know it. We may feel stressed, angry, or anxious and not realize that we are breathing shallowly because we're stuck in traffic or worried about something in the future.

Fortunately, you can hop in and take control of your respiratory system and help bring your body back to homeostasis. The oxygen is critical, obviously, but part of the reason we need to breathe deeply is for detoxification and elimination of wastes, especially carbon dioxide.

Have you ever wondered where weight goes when you lose it? Research has found that some of the weight is expelled through water and some through heat, but a big portion of it is eliminated by your breath. Cesar Millan is the Dog Whisperer, but we are all, in fact, fat whisperers.

Breathing deep is powerful. But it's a tough state of affairs because we have to relearn how to breathe again. I say relearn because there was a time when you did it perfectly. If you ever see a peaceful baby breathing, their belly is rising high with each inhale and sinking in with each exhale.

If I'm at a live event and ask an audience member to demonstrate how to breathe deeply, the first thing that happens is their shoulders shoot straight up when they inhale. Funny, I didn't know your lungs and diaphragm are in your shoulders.

This is a result of habitual chest-breathing. You're just filling the store window display of your lungs and not fully exercising them and filling them with air.

To regain your ability to breathe like a pro, try this:

- Sit up straight in a comfortable position, with your head facing forward and your shoulders relaxed. You can close your eyes if you like, but it's not necessary.
- Place one hand on your belly and rest the other hand on your lap.
- Now, on your first inhale, you're going to think about filling your belly and lungs with air from the bottom up like pouring water into a container.
- Keeping your shoulders relaxed, breathe in deeply through your nose, filling your belly with air as you feel it expanding right in your hand. Fill your lungs to the very tip-top (while keeping your shoulders relaxed), then hold all of that energizing air in for 2 seconds.
- Now breathe out through your nose as you empty your belly and lungs of every drop of air. You can feel your belly collapsing right under your hand. Get out every drop and be empty so that you can be filled again with something better. Hold everything out for a count of two.
- Now, again, take a deep breath in, filling your belly and lungs with air from the bottom up like pouring water into a container.
- Repeat all steps for five complete rounds of deep inhales and exhales and see how you feel.

This can be extended for several more rounds as a highly beneficial breathing meditation, but just a few rounds of focused breathing can instantly change your physiology. This is a really powerful and important practice because you're learning how to instantly guide how your body feels. You can flip on your parasympathetic nervous system at will, and even be able to be more in control of your thoughts.

It's said that your mind is the kite, and your breath is the string. Where your breathing goes, your mind will tend to follow. Short, shallow breaths are connected to stress and anxiety. Deep, rhythmic breaths are connected to relaxation and control. This is why your original design has put the ability to go on manual breathing in your hands. No matter what's going on around you, and what you may have perceived as a threat, you have the ability to control how you respond, and you can always take your power back if you choose to do so.

Breathe deep, relax, and remember how powerful you are to change your state.

MIND FULL OF WHAT?

Another valuable strategy for meditation is *mindfulness* meditation. There are entire books written on the subject, but I'll give you the brief summary: Be . . . Here . . . *Now!*

Most of the time our thoughts are scurrying off into the future thinking about all of the things that we could and need to do . . . or off in the past thinking about the way things went or how they could have gone differently. Very rarely are we in the present moment, in our bodies, and really taking in life.

You can use mindfulness meditations to get back in your body, be more present, and not let time go by on things that don't even exist. As it's said, the past is a memory, the future is a dream, and the present is really the gift.

Getting in and using your senses is a great way to practice mindfulness meditations. Have you ever wondered why our culture has become obsessed with chefs and cooking shows? Of course, we love to eat. But it's the personalities of the chefs that we get connected with. When top chefs are doing their thing, it's like a deep meditation to them. The smells of the herbs, the sounds of the entrée sizzling on the grill, the texture of the food as they chop, dice, and slice it, the taste (oh, the taste!) as they sample to see if it meets their delight, and the sight of it all with the finished product elegantly displayed on the plate.

It truly is a meditative experience if you tune into it. That's what the best chefs do, and their personalities speak volumes because of it.

You can turn just about anything into a sensory-filled mindfulness meditation. Mindfulness is really about noticing and tuning in to things in the here and now.

While walking, you can notice the feel of the ground under your feet, or even breathe deeply, syncing your breath with your steps. You can tune in and be more mindful while you're eating, while you're talking to a friend (instead of thinking about what you're going to say, actually fully and completely listen to them), while taking a shower or a bath, while exercising, while having sex, while cleaning the house, and on and on. Really, anything you do can be more meditative. You'll be changing the way your brain operates and improving the health and well-being of your body, and by increasing your parasympathetic tone, you'll be setting yourself up for a lot more really great sleep.

What meditation truly does is give you the uncanny ability to focus. This directly affects sleep because when it's time to sleep, your focus should be on, well, sleep. You can take your focus and put it on what you want, instead of the bazillion other things that your mind can jump around to. Meditation is a skill, a tool, and a necessity to help you relax. So, now that we know the power of meditation, and have a sample breathing meditation and mindfulness practice to start with, here are a couple of additional tips to get the most out of your practice to improve your sleep and your brain, starting now.

PRIME TIME

One of the best times for meditation is when you're already close to the alpha and theta brain waves. This would be as soon as you wake up in the morning, or right before bed at night. As the American Academy of Sleep Medicine research showed, meditating in the morning is proven to help test subjects sleep at night. You're creating a conscious neuro-pathway to relaxation, a buffer against stress, and a profound sense of presence that will help you sleep better in the evening.

Start your own meditation practice beginning tomorrow morning (or right now if you're an A-player!). We hear all the time about unhealthy habits, but this is a *healthy* habit you can create to benefit your life in numerous areas. As little as 5 to 10 minutes to start your day will have a cumulative effect on your energy, focus, and ability to sleep smarter.

If you ever find yourself in a situation where you wake up too soon and have trouble going back to sleep, simply lie in your bed and practice a breathing meditation to put your brain into the alpha and/or theta state to mimic some of the benefits of the sleep you would normally be missing out on.

This is an incredible resource to have at your disposal when you need it.

It's all about having tools and strategies to utilize in our day-to-day lives. Meditation can help rejuvenate your body and mind, supplement your sleep, and improve your performance. If you need help with some additional meditation techniques, I have some for you in the bonus resource guide at sleepsmarterbook.com/bonus, plus some Power Tips below to help your mind and body recover when you're in a pinch.

◇ ◇ ◇ ◇

CALM IT DOWN
POWER TIP #1

If you decide to meditate at night to help you wind down for sleep, try doing it *before* you get into the bed, not while you're in bed. Again, the neuro-association you want to have with your bed is sleep (and sex if you're too sexy for this party), and that's it. You can sit by your bedside and meditate for a few minutes, then slide your way into bed for a great night's sleep.

CALM IT DOWN
POWER TIP #2

Use guided meditations to help you get acclimated when you're first starting out. They can be really helpful for extremely busy-minded people because your attention goes to the instructions along the way. Try out the guided meditations in the bonus resource guide.

CALM IT DOWN
POWER TIP #3

If you do want to use a simple meditation/mindfulness practice to help you fall asleep while lying in bed, try this:

- Lie peacefully on your back with a comfortable pillow to support your head if you need one.
- Take a deep breath, breathing in for 5 seconds, holding for 5 seconds,

then breathing out for 5 seconds, and holding out for 5 seconds. Do this sequence three times.

- Now shift your focus to breathing and circulating that oxygen to your toes. Visualize the air coming in through your nose then traveling down to your toes, and then back out (following the same breathing count above).

- Next, move your attention to your feet. Breathe in through your nose and circulate the air to your feet following the same breathing count above (5 seconds in, 5 seconds hold, 5 seconds out, 5 seconds hold).

- Next, move your attention to your ankles, then your shins, then your knees, then your thighs, going all the way up your body until you gently drift away. You have to experiment to find out what works best for you. Give this one a try anytime you like.

CALM IT DOWN
POWER TIP #4

If you've found that you are consistently waking up in the middle of the night, there could be a couple of potential causes. The most obvious culprit is abnormal hormone cycles. As we've discussed in previous chapters, optimizing your hormones through smart nutrition, exercise, and following the tips in this book is key to setting your hormones back on track. Another issue could be an unknown or unresolved sleep apnea. It can be sort of like a really, really weak person is choking you—not anything to blatantly hurt you, but just enough to annoy you and wake you up. Losing weight is key here, as you know, but you may want to work with a physician to get this checked out.

A few other issues to consider are low blood sugar (as we discussed in Chapter 13), problems in the gastrointestinal tract (as we discussed in Chapter 7), and (a big one) psychological stress. With all of the stressors surrounding us today, it can be overwhelming for just about any of us. Having a smart meditation practice and working on the things that you may be putting off could be a big key to significantly dropping your stress load.

Oftentimes psychological stress results from things we know we "need to do" or haven't let go of. Maybe it's working on a relationship you really want, or maybe it's letting another one go. Maybe it's working on a new job skill you really need, or maybe it's letting go of a job that doesn't suit you. Either way, if it's important to you, you've got to take action on doing what you've got to do. It doesn't all have to be in one day, but make a commitment to take at least a tiny action in that direction every day. That tiny bit of consistency can do wonders for your psychological well-being. If it's building a better relationship, you have to make a study of it. If it's doing better in your finances, you have to make a study of it. If it's improving your health and wellness, you have to make a study of it. Read a little each day, listen to audiobooks or podcasts, or regularly go to meet-ups and events to help you continue to make progress on cultivating the life you really want. Being fulfilled instead of freaked out is probably a lot closer than you know.

CALM IT DOWN
POWER TIP #5

There can be several reasons why our sleep gets interrupted from time to time, but the most significant thing to do is to not sweat it too much. Stacking the conditions in your favor using the Sleep Smarter strategies will help to radically improve the quality of the sleep that you *do* get and help to make your sleep more valuable and consistent. Of course, we want to make sure that you're not in a chronic state of sleep deprivation, but worrying about whether you're getting enough sleep on occasion, and stressing out over it, isn't helping anybody.

If your sleep happens to be interrupted, meditation and relaxation techniques can be very helpful. If you can simply lie in bed, stay relaxed, and think positive thoughts (even smile and be happy to be alive!), then go ahead and stay in bed. However, if you're still working on improving yourself and find that you are agitated and frustrated, then by all means give yourself permission to get out of bed and journal or read (with the right kind of lighting we covered in previous chapters to keep cortisol low). There's no need to create a negative neuro-association to your sleeping environment. You may find that you get sleepy again while reading and drift off. There is even some evidence that segmented sleep has been a part of human evolution. Segmented sleep is essentially going to bed early in the evening and sleeping 3 to 4 hours, waking up for an hour or two, then returning back to sleep for another 3 to 4 hours until morning. Though this might not be ideal for most people, it's another thing to put your mind at ease and know that you are okay.

CALM IT DOWN
POWER TIP #6

There are also more "active" forms of meditation that you can do to see many of the same benefits without sitting in one place. The *Journal of Health Psychology* published a study demonstrating that doing a daily qigong practice (pronounced *chee-gong*) for just 1 month was enough to increase sleep duration and other factors of psychological well-being. Qigong is a more than 4,000-year-old form of meditation and energy practice involving controlled breathing and movement exercises. It's growing rapidly in popularity today as more and more studies are advocating its benefits.

Another study published in the *International Journal of Neuroscience* found that a 6-week qigong practice improved the sleep quality and walking ability of patients with Parkinson's disease. The advantages just go on and on. You can check out my favorite qigong practice in the bonus resources as well.

Tai chi is often described as "meditation in motion," and it's another excellent practice to consider. A study conducted at the University of California, Los Angeles, on 112 healthy older adults with moderate sleep complaints found that 16 weeks of tai chi improved the quality and duration of sleep significantly more than the control group. So, whether it's a breathing meditation, guided meditation, or movement-based meditation like these, take action to uncover a practice that works for you. The benefits are outstanding, and it only takes a few minutes a day.

CHAPTER 17

USE SMART SUPPLEMENTATION

M any people look to supplements to help them sleep, but they come with a huge caveat. Ideally, you *first* need to address the lifestyle issues that are actually causing the sleep problem. If you jump to taking drugs or supplements, then you'll just be treating a symptom and increase the likelihood that you'll develop a dependency on something that can harm you long term.

So, focus on the lifestyle stuff in this book first. Then, if you want, you can respectfully add a natural sleep aid, too. I'm going to share with you four of the more gentle-to-moderate aids. Let's get started with the most time-tested sleep aid of all:

Chamomile: This herb has been used for thousands of years to treat everything from skin disorders to heart disease to inflammation. Today, numerous studies are proving the true efficacy of this ancient plant. For example, a study highlighted in *Molecular Medicine Reports* showed that chamomile flavonoids have significant anti-inflammatory properties and trigger COX-2 enzyme activity that reduces physical pain. The study also asserts that chamomile can be used as a mild sedative and sleep inducer.

The sedative effects appear to be due in large part to a particular flavonoid called *apigenin*. This compound is abundant in chamomile tea, and it binds to certain GABA receptors in the brain, naturally calming nervous system activity. Again, because it's a natural compound found in foods and medicinal herbs, it's going to tend to have additional health benefits, rather than a page full of potential negative side effects. Apigenin has also been found to be a very potent anti-cancer compound. Research published in the *International Journal of Oncology* and the journal *Pharmaceutical Research* identified that apigenin is protective against a wide variety of cancers (including cancers of the breast, digestive tract, skin, and prostate) and has high selectivity against cancer cells as opposed to noncancerous cells.

Chamomile has been used historically as a sleep aid, but now our modern testing methods are proving its efficacy for this and many other health benefits. What studies show is that chamomile can help calm the nervous system, relax muscles, and set you up for a better night's sleep when you need it.

Chamomile is an excellent tea to have before bed. Simply have a standard-size cup of tea with an organic, prepacked chamomile tea bag, and you'll be good to go.

Kava kava: This is actually the national drink of the beautiful island of Fiji. Kava kava is well known for its sedative properties and is commonly used to treat sleeplessness and fatigue. A 2004 study published in *Human Psychopharmacology* also found that 300 milligrams of kava kava may improve mood and cognitive performance. Several additional studies show that it's effective for reducing the signs and symptoms of anxiety (which is definitely an anti-sleep state to be in).

The most important sleep-related data on kava kava demonstrates that it may help to improve sleep quality and decrease the amount of time needed to fall asleep. Preparing a cup of kava kava tea can be part of a relaxing evening ritual.

Valerian: This traditional herb is the strongest of the three herbs I recommend and a moderate sedative. It's indicated for individuals who have a difficult time falling asleep, and it also promotes uninterrupted sleep. The root of the valerian plant is used as medicine and pressed into fresh juice or freeze-dried to form a powder.

For tea, you can use a prepackaged tea bag or simply pour 1 cup of boiling water over 1 teaspoon (2 to 3 grams) of dried root, steep for 5 to 10 minutes, strain the tea, and enjoy. There are also tinctures and dried powder supplement capsules of valerian as well as the previous two medicinal herbs.

5-HTP, GABA, and L-tryptophan: I bundled all three of these together because they are not the ideal choices, due to the fact that they're not natural herbal preparations like the previous three. These are isolated chemicals, and they can be helpful if intently monitored and used with caution.

5-HTP is a neurotransmitter precursor to serotonin. In our bodies, as you well know from previous chapters, serotonin gets converted into melatonin (the get-good-sleep hormone). In a study compiled by the University of Maryland Medical Center, people who took 5-HTP went to sleep quicker and slept more deeply than those who took a placebo. Researchers recommend 200 to 400 milligrams at night to stimulate serotonin, but it may take 6 to 12 weeks to be fully effective.

GABA is an important neurotransmitter in the central nervous system. In fact, it is the major inhibitory neurotransmitter in the brain. Therefore, it blocks the action of excitatory brain chemicals. Some people swear by the sedating effects of GABA to help manage stress. If GABA is of interest to you, 500 milligrams in the evening is a good place to start. Also, consider looking into the GABA precursors picamilon and phenibut.

L-tryptophan is actually the precursor to 5-HTP. Although you can't get 5-HTP in food, there are several foods that are rich in tryptophan, like turkey, chicken, pumpkin, sunflower seeds, collard greens, and sea veggies. Although these foods can be part of a healthy diet, the trace amounts of tryptophan found in them may not be enough to get the effects you're looking for. L-tryptophan is a simple over-the-counter supplement you can use in addition to what you get from your diet. It can ideally be taken 90 minutes before bed.

These, like all other supplements, will influence people differently. One supplement might be a miracle for one person that helps them reestablish their sleeping cycle, while for someone else it may cause them to have crazy dreams or even feel groggier in the morning. Bottom line: It's unique to you whether something is going to be helpful or not. This goes for food, supplements, and even exercise. You have to experiment to find out what is the most intelligent, safest, and most effective long-term choice for you.

THE MELATONIN MISTAKE

You will notice that I didn't include melatonin in the discussion above. This has become a very popular supplement as of late, with all of our society's sleeping issues. Many experts agree that melatonin supplementation can be very effective for *some* people. But what's critical to understand about melatonin is that it is an actual hormone you're taking. And just like any other hormone therapy, such as testosterone therapy or estrogen therapy, it comes with a greater risk of side effects and potential problems.

One of the main issues with melatonin supplementation is that it can potentially down-regulate your body's natural ability to utilize melatonin on its own. A study published in the *Journal of Biological Rhythms* discovered that faulty timing or large doses of melatonin can cause desensitization of melatonin receptors. Essentially, you can start shutting down your body's ability to even use melatonin at all.

Many people who've consistently taken melatonin notice that over time they've had to take more and more. And still, according to board-certified sleep specialist Michael J. Breus, PhD, their sleep quality really isn't necessarily better. In regards to melatonin, he says, "Remember, it's a hormone, not a vitamin." So, unless you want to chance creating a dependency or shutting down your body's ability to use melatonin, I'd say avoid it or at least try other things first.

Taking precursors to melatonin can be a few degrees safer, but still, a word of caution: The best way to use a sleep-regulating supplement is in a short-term period to establish a normal sleep pattern, or to reestablish a normal sleep pattern after a time zone change from travel or a time change due to daylight saving time.

Do safe, smart, natural things first, then only bring the supplements in to "supplement" the good things you're already doing.

◇ ◇ ◇ ◇

SUPPLEMENTATION
POWER TIP #1

It can't be stressed enough that all the other strategies in this book are recommended before supplementation. In nature, you would not see compounds like these anywhere. They typically have only a few decades of testing (if that) versus the thousands upon thousands of years that humans have been on the planet. Think about it. Your body has an ancient, infinitely intelligent design; then in comes a chemical isolate made at the science lab last week, and things might not go according to plan. There are some brilliant scientists and innovators making progress in supplementation and medicine that can be lifesaving, but please, never mistake a product in a capsule for being real food.

SUPPLEMENTATION
POWER TIP #2

Find the right dose for you. Some companies recommend dosages of their products that are often too low or too high for certain individuals. For example, if someone were to use melatonin (though it's not recommended), 150 micrograms for men or 100 micrograms for women would be the ideal place to start. Yet, a common dosage you'll find with some melatonin supplements can be as much as 3,000 micrograms! Height, weight, gut health, stress levels, inflammation, and more are all factors that play into how much of a supplement would be ideal for you. The best advice is to start low and work your way up, unless you are 100 percent certain in what you are doing.

SUPPLEMENTATION
POWER TIP #3

Don't mix sleep aids with alcohol. By mixing the two together, you can relax muscles too much, stop breathing, and find yourself waking up like Bruce Willis in *The Sixth Sense*. (Spoiler alert: He was dead and didn't know it.) Seriously, taking any sleeping aid (be it medication or a supplement) along with alcohol is a really bad idea. Be smart, be safe, and don't talk to the kid who says, "I see dead people."

CHAPTER 18

BE EARLY TO RISE

We talked at length in Chapter 2 about the benefits of sunlight in helping us get better sleep. To take it a step further, it's not the sunlight alone, but waking up during the early part of the day that sets the template for a great night's sleep.

According to psychiatrist and psychotherapist Tracey Marks, MD, "Going to sleep early and waking early syncs the body clock with the earth's natural circadian rhythms, which is more restorative than trying to sleep while the sun's up."

It may seem totally ironic that getting up early can help you sleep better at night, but this goes back to the fact that humans have certain patterns of sleep and wakefulness that we've only found a way to override within the last 100 years. There was a time, not that long ago in our history, that humans were prey and in tremendous danger if they were rummaging around at night.

It's often forgotten that humans are not nocturnal creatures, so let me give you a little proof to remind you:

- Our eyesight sucks in the darkness. Wild predators like lions have many more rods in their eyes that enable them to see better at night.

You can't see them, but they can see you = You're invited to dinner (but not as a guest).

- We don't have a very strong sense of smell either. Sure, you can smell the lady walking past you at the gym wearing far too much perfume (what is she trying to cover up anyway?), but nocturnal animals like the opossum can smell trouble from a mile out.
- We also can't hear well enough to navigate the darkness. A small noise from hundreds of feet away can perk up the ears of a gray fox. They can't see as well as other nocturnal animals, but their keen sense of hearing allows them to hunt and avoid danger at night.

Humans have amazing senses that are really accentuated during the day. This allows us to see vivid colors and beautifully blend together our other senses to understand our environment like no other creature can.

The invention of the light bulb helped to brighten our world and enabled us to innovate, grow, and create better communities. Yet the use of artificial light has morphed into an addiction that has seen our sleeping hours and health plummet to all-time lows. Truly, what good is innovation if we don't have our health to enjoy it?

You might think, "Well, we're not out in the wild anymore anyway. Time for a Netflix all-night marathon. Woohoo!" It's true that we're not out in the wild anymore, and our modern amenities do make life nice and comfy. Yet it's also true that your genetics haven't changed much from those of your ancestors who lived closer to nature. Genetic adaptations can take thousands of years. And, unless you're a character from the *Twilight* series, you just don't have that kind of time.

Humans, as well as other organisms, have evolved to adjust to predictable patterns of light and darkness. These patterns establish our internal clocks and hormonal cycles every day of our lives. Once artificial light stepped into the picture, it effectively varied the length of our days. The result, as we've discussed, is that the average person's sleep quality has dramatically decreased, and our body clocks are out of order as sleep and wake times constantly vary from one night to the next.

The lack of consistency may be one of the biggest issues of all. The irregular sleeping hours prevent your brain from settling into a pattern, creating a state of perpetual jet lag. It's not just *how* you sleep, but *when* you sleep, that helps to create the best version of you. It's critical to create a smart sleep schedule in our world today, and this starts with getting our buns up in the morning.

BEING PART OF THE EARLY RISER CLUB HAS BENEFITS

In 2008, a study from the University of North Texas found that students who identified themselves as morning people earned significantly higher grades. In fact, the early risers had a full grade point higher than the night owls in the study with a 3.5 to 2.5 GPA respectively. Waking up earlier obviously isn't the only factor in getting good grades, but it's definitely a correlation to take notice of. A better GPA could mean better career opportunities and bigger levels of success overall.

Speaking of career opportunities, research published in the *Journal of Applied Social Psychology* showed that early birds are more proactive than evening people, and so they tend to do well in business. The study went on to state that morning people also anticipate problems better and minimize them more effectively. This is a huge leverage point in business today as everything is changing so fast.

It's not that people who identify themselves as early risers are better people, or better at everything, for that matter. Other studies suggest that night-lovers tend to be smarter and more creative than morning types, have a better sense of humor, and can be more outgoing in some instances. The big issue, according to the *Harvard Business Review*, is that night owls are out of sync with the typical corporate schedule and miss out on critical opportunities more often because their timing is off.

So, whether you identify yourself as a morning person or a night owl, you can do amazing things with your life. I just want to ensure that you have the greatest advantage possible, and that your health is up to par to create the life you really want. This leads to the reality that your health is radically improved when you're honoring your body's natural hormonal clock. Humans are designed to be up during the day and sleeping at night. Being a night owl is a new idea, and you're not literally an owl anyway.

NOT A MORNING PERSON?

Some people just love getting up early in the morning to take advantage of the day. It's a very empowering feeling to have accomplished so much long before other people have even gotten out of bed. Various studies show that morning people tend to exhibit character traits like optimism, satisfaction, and conscientiousness. Getting started on your work goals by 8:00 a.m. gives you an extra sense of optimism in and of itself, whereas by 4:00 p.m., you've had seven minor problems that have tried to throw you off your course.

Again, being a night owl is a new idea that has only been possible in recent human history. This is a trained behavior that, like it or leave it, is influencing your health and the results in your life.

If you firmly believe you are a night owl and want to make the switch to get your circadian rhythms, hormones, and priorities in order, there are simple steps to do it.

Leo Babauta from the wildly popular Web site *Zen Habits* recommends using a gradual method when changing your sleep schedule. Rather than making the decision to suddenly get up at 6:00 a.m. when you normally get up at 8:00 a.m., take gradual 15-minute increments off your wake-up time until you get to your desired destination.

This is a much more graceful way to do it. Oftentimes when people decide to get up early, they throw their sleep cycles into such a shocked state that they're more tired and irritated, plus they've created a neuro-association between more pain and waking up early. This causes them to burn through their willpower within days and revert to their old habits before they know it.

If your goal is to wake up at 6:00 a.m. and you are currently getting up at 8:00 a.m., set your alarm for 7:45 a.m. instead. Do that for a few days, then move to 7:30 a.m., then move to 7:15 a.m., and so on. This will allow your body to adapt to the new schedule in a much healthier and sustainable way.

So how do you resist the urge to just hit the snooze button and forfeit your commitment to getting up?

Leo Babauta offered these three suggestions, and I have to say, they're pretty brilliant:

1. **Get excited.** The night before, think of one thing you'd like to do in the morning that excites you. It could be something you want to write, or a new yoga routine, or meditation, or something you'd like to read, or a work project that has you fired up. In the morning, when you wake up, remember that exciting thing, and that will help motivate you to get up.

2. **Jump out of bed.** Yes, jump out of bed. With enthusiasm. Jump up and spread your arms wide as if to say, "Yes! I am alive! I'm ready to tackle the day with open arms and the gusto of a driven maniac." Seriously, it works.

3. **Put your alarm across the room.** If it's right next to you, you'll hit the snooze button. So put it on the other side of the room, so you'll have to get up (or jump up) to turn it off. Then, get into the habit of going straight to the bathroom to pee once you've turned it off. Once you're done peeing, you're much less likely to go back to bed. At this point, remember your exciting thing. If you didn't jump out of bed, at least stretch your arms wide and greet the day.

Putting your alarm across the room is also ideal to reduce your amount of EMF exposure, as we discussed in Chapter 12. The EMFs from electronic devices disrupt the communication between the cells in your body, and they're obviously stronger if they're plugged in right next to you. It's not a smart move to sleep with any electronic devices near your body, so don't do it.

Here's one more bonus suggestion to beat the urge to go back to bed, and instead energize your body to be ready to take on the day: *Wake up your senses.*

When you get out of bed, get your senses stimulated with something good. A common thing to do is to get that coffee or tea brewing and drink it. The smell, taste, and touch are all enlivening for your senses.

I'm a huge advocate of drinking a big glass or two of water first thing in the morning. I call this an inner bath. This will replenish your hydration levels that went down while you were sleeping, help your body to clear out metabolic waste products, and give you a sensory stimulation to help wake up your body. You can also take a regular bath or shower, too, to get you going. Or use more of your senses by turning on some good music and opening the curtains to let in the natural light. There are so many things that will automatically get your mind and body stimulated when you're exposed to them. Try these things out and start your day with real momentum.

By waking up early, you start helping your endocrine system link up with the diurnal patterns of the Earth. Get up when the sun rises. It might be challenging at first, but after less than a couple of weeks, your body will adapt to that pattern and you'll feel much more rested and refreshed when you wake up. You can break the old pattern of being up at night "tired and wired" by being early to rise and having a natural release of cortisol, then going to bed earlier and taking advantage of the natural release of melatonin. A quote from one of my son's favorite books, the epic masterpiece *Winnie-the-Pooh*: "For early to bed, and early to rise will make a bear happy, and healthy, besides."

◇ ◇ ◇ ◇

EARLY TO RISE
POWER TIP #1

Go to bed within 30 minutes of the same time each night and wake up at the same time each day. Many people in our modern world try to "catch up" on sleep and sleep in on the days that they don't have to get up for work. By throwing off your sleep schedule like this, you'll usually find that you're more tired than you want to be on your off days, and really dreading getting out of bed once Monday rolls around. Remember, a consistent sleep schedule is important for your health.

Try to avoid staying up much later just because you're off the next day. Actually go to bed and get up so that you can *use* that day to do the things you want. I promise you, Netflix does still work during the daytime, and you can get a mini-marathon in without the same side effects you'll experience if you'd stayed up all night.

To stay within your body's desired sleep pattern, you don't have to go to bed at exactly 10:02 p.m. each night, but do your best to make it within 30 minutes of what your ideal sleep time is.

EARLY TO RISE
POWER TIP #2

Leo Babauta's gradual method works on the other side of getting optimized sleep, too: getting to bed earlier and getting more "money time" sleep. As we saw in Chapter 6, you will get even more hormonal benefits, enzymatic repair and activity, and overall physical and mental rejuvenation by getting to bed earlier and capitalizing on sleep between the hours of 10:00 p.m. and 2:00 a.m.

If you've been habitually staying up until 1 o'clock in the morning, suddenly deciding to go to sleep 2 hours earlier could end up being a rocky transition if you try to do it all in one night. Instead, utilize the gradual method, also referred to as *advancing the internal clock*, to gradually move your bedtime up a little bit earlier until the desired bedtime is reached. If your goal is to be in bed by 11:00 p.m. and you're currently getting to bed at 1:00 a.m., simply move your bedtime up by 15 minutes every couple of days until you hit the goal you really want. Of course, you can rip the Band-Aid off and go *early to bed and early to rise* cold turkey, but this is a much more graceful way for you to get there and to enjoy the process of getting better sleep that much faster.

CHAPTER 19

USE BODYWORK THAT WORKS

In a study on chronic pain sufferers published by the *International Journal of Neuroscience*, it was found that, in addition to decreased long-term pain, test subjects receiving massage therapy experienced improved sleep and an increase in serotonin levels.

We all know that massage feels great. But many of us underestimate just how powerful it can be for great sleep. Massage is like a secret key to unlocking your sympathetic (fight-or-flight) nervous system and activating your parasympathetic (rest-and-digest) nervous system. When you add in the clinically proven benefits on serotonin production, oxytocin, and reduction of cortisol, it's no wonder that massage can be so helpful for gliding off to dreamland.

How do you feel after getting a great massage? You probably don't feel like running a 5-K or cleaning up your house; chances are you don't feel like doing much of anything except relaxing. Everything is calm, cool, and peaceful. Things that would normally bother you, don't; your patience is higher; and you might have a slight joker-ish smile on your face as you look at other people and think, "Why so serious?"

Even though we know that massage is a great remedy for stress, people are often shocked to find out the other benefits that massage can deliver.

Here are just a few of the notable benefits:

- Normalization of blood pressure
- Reduction of inflammatory cytokines
- Reduced pain
- Improved mobility
- Improved symptoms of anxiety and depression
- Reduction in migraines and headaches
- Improved digestion and elimination
- Reduction of stress hormones
- Improved immune system function

As you might guess from reading about the significance of immune system health, the immune-massage connection is particularly important.

A study led by Mark Hyman Rapaport, MD, chair of the department of psychiatry and behavioral sciences at Emory University School of Medicine in Atlanta, demonstrated that over a 5-week period of time, weekly massage showed substantial neuroendocrine and immune system benefits. Some of the results seen in the study were an improvement in the number of lymphocytes (white blood cells that help manage the immune system), a decrease in cortisol, a decrease in arginine vasopressin (a hormone believed to play a role in aggression), and a reduction in cytokines linked to inflammation.

The question is, with so many benefits related to massage, why aren't more people utilizing it?

RUBBING HISTORY

Massage has a deep, rich history dating back over 5,000 years. Archeological evidence of massage therapy has been found in many ancient civilizations including those in China, Egypt, India, Japan, Rome, and Greece. Throughout time, massage has been used as an effective healing tool. The person often referred to as the father of modern medicine, the Greek physician Hippocrates, said, "The physician must be experienced in many things, but assuredly in rubbing."

As time passed and we moved into the 20th century, massage was still being used in hospitals by nurses to help ease patients' pain and help them sleep. However, around the 1970s, massage in the medical profession began to fall quickly out of favor with the advent of much more powerful pain medication and tranquilizers.

Even still, the field of massage sprouted its own legs and began to grow as a form of therapy, particularly within the world of athletics. Only in recent years have well-conducted studies been done on the value of massage for other health benefits, and this coincided with popular culture starting to put a higher demand on massage. I bet you've noticed a whole lot more massage studios around town, haven't you?

At present day, approximately 10 percent of the US population is utilizing massage therapy at least on a semiconsistent basis. One of the big reasons it's growing in popularity is the experiential benefits on reducing stress and improving sleep (many people don't even make it off the massage table before they drift off to sleep).

One study monitoring brain activity found that massage actually increases delta brain waves. As you know from Chapter 16, delta brain waves are associated with complete relaxation and deep, regenerative sleep. This is yet another reason that bodywork shouldn't be a rare treat in your life; it should really be a necessity.

WHAT'S YOUR TYPE?

Many of the latest studies utilized Swedish massage, which is a technique where pressure is varied from light to vigorous and the muscles are rubbed with long, gliding strokes in the direction of blood returning to the heart. Swedish massage is awesome, though it's just one type of massage that can deliver a whole new world of value to your body and sleep.

Here are some of the other forms of massage and bodywork that have been shown to deliver many of the health-giving benefits we've been discussing:

Acupressure	Lomi lomi
Ayurvedic massage	Myofascial release
Craniosacral therapy	Reflexology

Shiatsu   Thai massage

Sports massage   Watsu

Stone massage

You'll notice that many of these forms of massage require another person, and that's what usually comes to mind when we think about massage. However, there are many forms of bodywork and self-massage that simply require you, your body (which you are hopefully with all the time), and maybe a few cool tricks to maximize your results.

A wonderful form of massage that can be done with a practitioner or on your own is acupressure massage. A comprehensive study conducted through the department of radiotherapy and oncology at San Gerardo Hospital in Monza, Italy, found that 60 percent of patients with sleep disorders had an improvement in sleep quality after at least 2 weeks of acupressure treatment. What was even more impressive is that 79 percent of cancer patients in the study had improvements in their sleep quality. But how does this work?

Acupressure (a blend of the words *acupuncture* and *pressure*) is a form of therapy that's been used for more than 2,000 years. According to researchers, there are specific places in your body where nerves relay signals to other organs and glands of the body if they are engaged. Acupressure is essentially a method of sending a signal to the body (by needle or other means) to "turn on" its own self-healing or regulatory mechanisms. It's not really radical to understand at all. We all know that every cell in our bodies is managed by a governing force that is our brain. Every cell, tissue, and organ can give and receive data across this information superhighway that is your body.

The acupressure point used in the study was HT 7, which is right under the palm of your hand near the edge of your wrist. In another, double-blind, placebo-controlled study on insomnia patients, manipulation of the HT 7 point over the course of the study increased urinary melatonin metabolites to normal levels. Basically, the researchers could see from the participants' tinkle that melatonin was doing its job in their bodies.

HT 7 ACUPRESSURE POINT ASSOCIATED WITH
IMPROVED SLEEP QUALITY

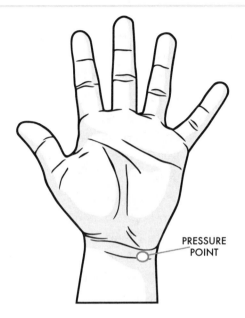

PRESSURE
POINT

There are many acupressure points on the human body that have been heavily researched. Working with a skilled practitioner and doing some research on your own would be a good idea if you want to learn more about them. Other forms of acupressure-based therapies to check out are EFT (Emotional Freedom Technique) and traditional acupuncture.

GET YOUR ROLL ON

At night, right before bed, is a great time to employ some bodywork and self-massage to deactivate your sympathetic nervous system.

On a popular episode of my show, *New York Times* bestselling author Kelly Starrett, DPT, told me that he's found a very specific form of bodywork that is also a powerful sleep aid. He said, "One of the biggest problems we have in society right now is people aren't very good at down-regulating. What we see is people getting into a constant sympathetic nervous system versus parasympathetic nervous system tug-of-war, and the sympathetic nervous system is turned all the way up to 60. We know that you can power up by drinking some coffee or chugging an energy drink and be ready to go, but show me how you can go (in reverse) from 60 to 0. One of the ways that we know makes a big difference is doing this very complex, very sophisticated thing called *gut smashing.*"

Dr. Starrett saying that it is complex is a little tongue-in-cheek because though its actions are complex, it's something that's incredibly easy to do. Strategically massaging your abdominal wall, or what he calls gut smashing, likely works in part by stimulating your vagus nerve. As we discussed in Chapter 7, your vagus nerve interfaces with your heart, lungs, and other organs on a pathway straight to your brain. And researchers at UCLA discovered that around 90 percent of the fibers in the vagus nerve carry information from your gut to your brain (and not the other way around). So, what goes on with your belly can, in essence, tell your brain and nervous system what to do. Here's how it's done:

Get yourself a ball that has a little give to it. Dr. Starrett recommends the inexpensive plastic balls you might find in a ball bin at a discount department store. You want a ball that's about the size of a soccer ball or kickball, and, again, it should have some give to it, so make sure it's not too full of air before you use it.

Now, get down on the floor and lay belly-down on the ball. Dr. Starrett says, "Spend 5 to 10 minutes 'ungluing' your abdominal musculature—just rolling back and forth, stopping where it's uncomfortable, contracting and relaxing, just breathing into that ball. It's safe and effective, and it triggers your parasympathetic system to turn on." After working with thousands of athletes and patients from all over the world, he says it's one of the most efficient ways to help your system down-regulate. You can check out a video with Dr. Starrett and world-renowned therapist Jill Miller demonstrating how to do this in the bonus resource guide at sleepsmarterbook .com/bonus.

So, whether it's Swedish massage, Thai massage, acupressure, gut smashing, myofascial release, or anything else, make it a mandate to get some bodywork in on a regular basis. We hold so much tension, stress, and inflammation in our bodies, and this is one time-tested way to get your body, mind, and sleep back in balance.

◇◇◇◇

BODYWORK
POWER TIP #1

Book yourself a massage this week. When's the last time you got a massage? If it's recently, I'd like to congratulate you. Right now, about 10 percent of the US population gets a massage regularly, and that number is growing fast. If you don't know of, or don't currently have the resources for a private massage therapist, then book an appointment at one of the national massage studios because they always have great deals for new clients. It would be the best idea ever to get yourself a monthly membership at one of these massage studios as well. It'll make sure that you're going in at least once a month, and it will also give you the ability to try different forms of massage and different therapists until you find one who clicks with you.

BODYWORK
POWER TIP #2

Give progressive muscle relaxation a shot. You might think that your muscles are relaxed, but they're probably not. Many of us hold in constant muscle tension where our muscles are slightly "on" even when we consciously believe that we are fully relaxed. To help combat this and truly relax those muscles, the best thing you can do is fully tense them up first. Sound strange?

Philip Gehrman, PhD, clinical director of Penn Medicine's behavioral sleep medicine program at the Penn Sleep Center in Philadelphia, says, "Progressive muscle relaxation is a relaxation exercise in which you systematically tense and then relax all the muscle groups of your body. It helps promote overall physical relaxation, which has a number of benefits on its own."

Basically, by fully contracting your muscles, you can elicit (and experience) a greater relaxation when you let go. This practice is used clinically to help reduce stress and improve sleep. Here's a sample of how it's done:

Lie down in a comfortable position and take a few deep breaths to begin the practice. Starting with your face, tense all the muscles either all at once or one at a time, which is even better. Hold each contraction for 5 to 10 seconds. Lift your eyebrows as high as possible, bring them down as low as possible, squeeze your eyes shut, tense your lips, cheeks, and jaw. Then totally let go and relax.

Next move to your shoulders and arms. Hold each contraction for 10 seconds from here on. Tense your shoulders, clench your fists tightly, and contract the muscles in your arms. After the 10 seconds, let them totally relax, feel the deeper relaxation, and wait a few seconds before moving on. Next, go to your chest and abdomen, then to your back, then to your hips and butt, and finish with your legs and feet, devoting a 10-second tense-and-relax session to each one for at least one round. You will likely notice a significant decrease in your stress level and greater relaxation in your body overall.

BODYWORK
POWER TIP #3

There are many other tools that you can use for self-massage at home, including foam rollers, tennis balls, lacrosse balls, and trigger point massage tools, just to name a few. And, of course, you have your own hands for self-massage, or a partner's hands if you know how to ask nicely. Make it a consistent part of your nightly ritual to get just a couple minutes of bodywork in to de-stress from the day.

CHAPTER 20

DRESS FOR THE OCCASION

Humans are unique in the fact that many of us get dressed up just to go to bed. We have special bed attire that we call pajamas, and it's just one of those words that's synonymous with comfiness. Go ahead and say it slowly and tell me it doesn't feel good. "Pajamas . . . Pajamas . . . "

Putting on your pj's can be like a mental trigger to relax and wind down for the day. You're getting out of your outer-world uniform and putting clothes on your body that make you feel safe, relaxed, and at home. The reality is, you're not just wearing clothes that only your inner circle of friends and family can see you in (unless you're going to a Pajama Jammy Jam), but you're also putting on clothes that will inherently affect the quality of your sleep.

As we covered in Chapter 5, thermoregulation is a critical aspect of managing sleep quality. Research shows that certain forms of insomnia are linked to faulty body temperature regulation and an inability to cool down enough to enter deeper stages of sleep. It's important to realize that your body is better at keeping itself warm than keeping itself cool, so you'll make it easier on yourself by wearing fewer and looser clothes to bed.

In a Dutch study, scientists had participants wear thermosuits to lower their skin temperature less than 1°C (without affecting core body temperature) to measure its impact on sleep. The study results showed that the participants didn't wake up as much during the night, and that the amount of time spent in stages three and four (deep sleep) had increased.

If you think that what you're wearing to bed doesn't matter, think again.

Now, I'm not saying that you have to freeze your tootsies off just to get better sleep, but I am saying that if you're used to dressing up like an Eskimo to hop in the sack, you might want to consider pulling off a layer or two.

If you live in a home where you can regulate the temperature, you're more fortunate than billions of other people on the planet. With that said, overdoing it on the warmth can result in you not feeling rested when you wake up, even if you slept the "right" amount of hours. If you have seven covers and an electric blanket, and you're dressed like you're going hunting, you just might be preventing your body from getting the most rejuvenating stages of sleep.

MIDNIGHT STRANGLER

The form and fit of your bedtime clothing is more significant than any fashion statement you can make. Wearing tight, restrictive clothing to bed is a huge sleep mistake you need to avoid. Clothing that is too tight can literally cut off the flow of your lymphatic system. Your lymphatic system is the cellular "waste management" system of your body, and an important part of your immune system. It transports and circulates extracellular fluid throughout your body, and you actually have 4 times more lymph fluid than you have blood.

When your lymphatic system gets cut off due to restrictive clothing, that extracellular fluid can start to pool in different places in your body, and real nastiness can ensue from there.

The most common culprit here is tight socks. You'll know your socks are probably too tight if, when you pull them off, you can still see the imprint of the socks perfectly on your skin. It's a nice party trick, but this is not good at all.

It's through the lymphatic system that toxic substances can move out of the body. If it's cut off in any way, it's like bending a water hose and blocking the water's ability to flow out. The water pressure will swell, and you can mess up your internal plumbing or worse.

In Chapter 5, I recommended that you keep the bedroom cool, but also wear a pair of warm socks if you tend to get cold easily. To remedy the problem of choking your ankles out while you sleep, simply opt for a pair of loose, fuzzy socks as your go-to choice. Many types of hiking socks have a looser fit, so that might be a good place to start.

Beyond the lower extremities, there could be an even bigger and more dangerous issue for women. This may come as a shock, but a 2009 study found that women who slept in their bras had a 60 percent greater risk for developing breast cancer.

Numerous studies are now confirming the link between breast cancer and habitual bra wearing. This doesn't mean you should throw your bras away, but it does mean that you need to be conscientious of this connection. When you take off your bra and see those indentions around your back, sides, shoulders, and breasts, that's a clear indication that you're cutting off lymphatic flow and circulation.

The lymph nodes and lymph function are a critical component in preventing the development of diseases, including breast cancer. Many women have been trained to wear their bras 24-7 for fear of what society will think, to avoid sagging breasts, or even to prevent back pain. Though these beliefs can become very real to an individual, the research shows that these worries are simply not valid.

A 15-year study involving more than 300 women concluded: "Medically, physiologically, anatomically, the breast does not benefit from being deprived of gravity." Overall, it was found that women who do not use bras developed more muscle tissue to naturally support their breasts and had greater nipple lift (in relation to their shoulders). Conversely, women who wore bras had actually accelerated breast sagging.

Again, this is contrary to a deeply ingrained public opinion, but it's actually based on sound science. Bras can make breasts look *amazing* while they're being worn. But if the breasts are constantly held weightless by the bra, they have very little opportunity to develop the ability to support themselves. It's just like any other body part: If you don't use it, it will atrophy.

Since our main focus here is improving your sleep, and improving your health as a result of it, at night while you're asleep is an obvious time to go bra free and cut your risk of major problems from wearing a bra 24 hours a day. We don't have to start up a Bra-a-holics Anonymous. But, if you want to get more information on the bra–breast cancer connection, check out the book *Dressed to Kill* by medical anthropologists Sydney Ross Singer and Soma Grismaijer.

As for the fellas, tight, restrictive clothing can cause less-than-desired results, too. Namely, the choice in underwear can potentially have a *huge* impact on reproductive health.

A study published in *Reproductive Toxicology* sought to test the validity of the commonly held (but often overlooked) notion that habitually wearing tight underwear can damage sperm. The test subjects were required to alternate from wearing tight-fitting briefs to loose-fitting boxer-type underwear at different points throughout the study, which lasted 3 months. The semen parameters tested were: sperm density, total number of sperm, total number of motile sperm, and total number of motile sperm per hour of abstinence. By the end of the study, the results showed conclusively that the semen parameters gradually *decreased* when the men wore tighter underwear and gradually *increased* when the men wore looser underwear.

This type of study simply affirms what we know about the biological function of the testes and, in particular, the cremaster muscle, whose function is to raise and lower the testes in order to regulate temperature for optimal spermatogenesis and survival of the sperm.

On a really enlightening episode of my show, biomechanist and bestselling author Katy Bowman, MS, shared insights about how our environment actually shapes our bodies. We tend to think that we get the shape of our bodies from exercise, diet, and genetics, but Katy disclosed how "cellular loads" that we're exposed to also shape our bodies as well. For example, the way you sit in a chair or stand creates a certain load that impacts everything from your head to your toes, and if you shift your body just one degree in any direction, it creates a completely different cellular experience. Habitually doing any movement (or lack of movement) will effectively influence the way your body is organized. And in this example, the habitual wearing of tight underwear changes the natural loads that would occur for the male reproductive bits.

Katy shared that it isn't just a problem for the testes, but the entire surrounding area and our health as a whole. She stated, "You get atrophy of a muscle, and then the circulation to a muscle goes down. The action of a muscle doesn't only accomplish a movement; there are movements of blood to local areas *around* a muscle based on a movement. So you don't just disable the muscle—you disable the circulation of blood and nutrients to the broader area."

As you can see, it's never just one cell, tissue, or organ that is affected. Your choices affect so much more because *you* are so much more. Your body is highly intelligent and sophisticated in its design, and nothing happens in isolation. The choices we make each day directly influence how our cells will respond. So, whether it's a choice in movement, food, sleep, or even the clothes that we wear, something is always going to result from it. And the power is always in your hands to determine what those results will look like.

SHOPPING WITH OUR EYES CLOSED

Have you ever heard the phrase "form over fashion"? It's the idea that what we wear should facilitate natural function, allow natural movement, and actually feel good (not just look good) on our bodies. In our culture we've been conditioned to wear some incredibly restrictive and even *painful* clothing for the sake of looking good, fitting in, or being fashionable.

Now, I'm not advocating that we can't look amazing and have incredible clothes to wear. Fashion has come a long way, so I say that we continue to more forward and not go back. (I mean, seriously, have you seen some of the stuff we used to wear? Parachute pants and bell-bottom jeans just look silly, and they were clearly a tripping hazard, too.) But understanding that the clothes we wear are also impacting our health is an important insight to have. We can wear and demand clothes that not only look good, but feel good as well.

Being an underwear model is a high-status job in our culture, as funny as it might sound. We want to look like the person in the ad, and to a lot of people, tight stuff just looks better. We can definitely rock some tighter clothes from time to time, but make it a habit to counterbalance things and let your body be free.

The best clothing for bed will be nonrestricting and hypoallergenic (both the fabric itself and how it's washed). I'm not saying you should wear one of those one-size-fits-all nightgowns that look like a bed sheet with a hole cut in the middle to stick your head through. Be comfortable, and get comfortable with your own body being freer. There are countless attractive options for bed attire if that's important to you. I'm just going to share the basics. Here are just a few options on what to wear to bed:

Men: Boxers, loose-fitting pajama bottoms, basketball shorts, basic T-shirt if you want, or go naked

Women: Boy shorts, your own or your significant other's T-shirt or boxers, flowing lingerie, yoga pants or "tights" that don't strangle your legs and hips, loose-fitting pajama bottoms, or go naked

BIRTHDAY SUIT

If you and your partner both sleep in the nude, you can reap the benefits of the feel-good hormone oxytocin. You can get these benefits from intimacy (like sleeping in the same bed), massage, sex, or simply cuddling; the skin-to-skin contact is all that's required. Oxytocin is a potent anti-stress hormone. It reduces the signs and symptoms of depression, combats the negative effects of cortisol, and helps regulate blood pressure. It's also been shown to decrease intestinal inflammation and improve gut motility as well. All the more reason to get as close as possible.

On top of all this is the obvious: More sex. As we covered in Chapter 9, an orgasm might just be nature's number one sleep aid.

◇ ◇ ◇ ◇

DRESS FOR THE OCCASION
POWER TIP #1

A 1991 Harvard study found that women who do not wear bras had half the risk of breast cancer compared to avid bra users. Take bedtime as an optimal opportunity to go bra free. This is a great start to improving your health and cutting down on your programmed bra dependency. For the guys, avoid wearing tight underwear to bed that keeps your testicles pressed against your body. You're potentially overheating your family jewels, and not allowing them to extend and retract based on a more natural temperature. Bedtime is a perfect time to wear something looser or to not wear anything at all.

DRESS FOR THE OCCASION
POWER TIP #2

When shopping for clothes, keep in mind the cellular loads (or lack thereof) that get created from the items you choose to wear. There are a lot more companies (including high fashion) that are creating clothing and shoes that help to support the normal, natural function of the human body while still looking fantastic. You can find several of these companies in the Sleep Smarter bonus resource guide at sleepsmarterbook.com/bonus, so make sure to check it out!

CHAPTER 21

GET GROUNDED

Since the beginning of time, humans have had a constant interaction with the earth. Our ancestors would come in contact with the earth's surface on a daily basis: walking, hunting, gathering food and water, communing, playing, relaxing, and more. Nearly everything they did required a connection with the earth.

Today, in our industrialized world, many people go days, weeks, or even longer without coming in contact with the surface of the Earth itself. We are cooped up in our homes or offices, spending more time indoors consuming technology and less time interacting with the source of all that technology. Sure, we may walk outside to get into our cars, but most of us wear nonconductive rubber-soled shoes that ensure our bodies never get that intimate connection. We rarely touch the ground, rarely touch a tree, and rarely touch the source that creates every cell in our bodies.

Scientists are discovering that this is having a huge impact on our health.

Overwhelming research is mounting that shows the impressive benefits the earth's electromagnetic surface has on the human body. We may not realize this, but the human body is highly conductive. We, like the earth, are running on electromagnetic energy. Our nervous system is like internal wiring that's transmitting information throughout our entire body. We're also made of minerals, and our tissues hold water, so we are very much like a walking, talking, conductive battery.

You've probably noticed that we can accumulate static electricity and "shock" someone who touches us. We all know not to stick a metal object into an outlet or we'll "short out" our system. Even in scary movies, one of the worst ways to go is having an electric device tossed into your bathtub while you're trying to exfoliate.

Bottom line: You may not be able to see it, but you are highly conductive. You give off and receive energy every second of every day. The misuse and misunderstanding of your body's electrical system is a catalyst for chronic health problems.

So, how does this relate to you, the earth, your health, and your sleep?

Currently, more than 90 percent of physician visits are for stress- and inflammatory-related issues. Stress and inflammation go hand in hand and are a huge undercurrent in the vast majority of diseases. Researchers at Emory University School of Medicine in Atlanta have also found that poor sleep quality is intimately related to inflammation. It may sound a little strange, but touching the earth may be the biggest key to eliminating our issues with chronic inflammation.

INFLAMMATION NATION

We now understand that the human body is conductive. Every tissue in the body carries a charge, and this is actually what allows many functions to happen. Inflammation, in particular, is a natural function facilitated by a type of white blood cell called a *neutrophil*. Neutrophils deliver reactive oxygen species (also known as free radicals) to the site of an injury or need. These free radicals carry a positive charge that will tear harmful bacteria apart and break apart damaged cells to create room for healthy cells to move in and repair tissues. Pretty cool, right?

Inflammation is not supposed to be a catastrophic thing. The real problem arises when free radical activity goes unchecked and some of those free radicals leak into the surrounding tissue and damage healthy cells. This is the real cause of inflammation, and most people are dealing with this at chronic levels on a day-to-day basis.

Every day you have cellular damage, simply by the nature of being alive. Damaged heart cells, liver cells, muscle cells, etc., all set off an oxidative burst of free radicals to address them. This is basic chemistry, featuring a *positive* charged event that needs to be neutralized.

All the rage in health and nutrition today has been centered on antioxidants. Antioxidants carry free electrons that neutralize free radicals and stop overly aggressive oxidation right in its tracks. Inflammation is reduced, and health is improved.

The reality is that you can eat foods that are high in antioxidants until you're blue in the face (from eating a lot of blueberries, of course), but this isn't going to swing the battle of oxidation in your favor as much as you think.

First of all, the antioxidants need to be in the right form, and conventional food processing techniques tend to strip the antioxidant potency from our food. Secondly, the dietary antioxidants have to withstand the digestive process, make their way through the gut lining, and hopefully find their way into your blood. Thirdly, dietary antioxidants have been found to pale in comparison to your body's own endogenous antioxidant capabilities. The ability of your liver to support production of the antioxidant *superoxide dismutase*, for example, is more potent than any antioxidant you can consume. The key is getting your body into the right state so that your organs and tissues can do the great job they already know how to do. Lastly, it's been discovered that the number one source of free electrons is actually the source where all of our food comes from: the earth itself.

Scientists have discovered that the earth's surface is brimming with free electrons that are readily absorbed by the human body when they come in contact with each other. This is known as an electron transfer. The effects of this electron transfer are being researched rigorously, and the impact on sports performance, healing, and overall health is shocking.

Researchers are calling this connection with the human body and the earth *grounding* or *earthing*.

A study published in the 2013 issue of the *Journal of Alternative and Complementary Medicine* showed that "grounding increases the surface charge on red blood cells and thereby reduces blood viscosity and clumping. Grounding appears to be one of the simplest and yet most profound interventions for helping reduce cardiovascular risk and cardiovascular events."

Wait, hold up. . . . Just getting in contact with the earth's surface can improve my blood and lower my risk of a heart attack?

Renowned cardiologist and bestselling author Stephen Sinatra, MD, had this to say: "Reduction in inflammation as a result of earthing has been documented with infrared medical imaging and with measurements of blood chemistry and white blood cell counts. The logical explanation for the anti-inflammatory effects is that grounding the body allows negatively charged antioxidant electrons from the earth to enter the body and neutralize positively charged free radicals at sites of inflammation. Flow of electrons from the earth to the body has been documented."

As for stress, it's been confirmed that earthing has a measurable impact on stress reduction by shifting the autonomic nervous system from sympathetic to parasympathetic dominance, improving heart rate variability, and normalizing muscle tension. In a study published in the *Journal of Environmental and Public Health*, researchers found that when test subjects were grounded, there was a "rapid activation of the parasympathetic nervous system and corresponding deactivation of the sympathetic nervous system." As you know from previous chapters, the importance of being able to shift out of the constant barrage of fight-or-flight of the sympathetic nervous system and into the parasympathetic,

ELECTRON TRANSFER FROM THE EARTH TO HUMAN TISSUES

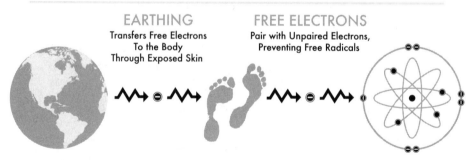

EARTHING
Transfers Free Electrons
To the Body
Through Exposed Skin

FREE ELECTRONS
Pair with Unpaired Electrons,
Preventing Free Radicals

rest-and-digest system is of the utmost importance for your sleep and health overall.

I wouldn't have thought that something as simple as coming in contact with the earth would be so powerful if the data weren't so thick. For a comprehensive understanding of earthing and its benefits, be sure to check out the bonus resource guide at sleepsmarterbook.com/bonus.

For now, just don't be the last person to make this connection, and utilize the free, health-giving resource you have right outside your front door.

WHAT ABOUT SLEEP?

A study published in 2004 looked at the biological effects of grounding the human body during sleep as measured by cortisol levels and subjective reporting of sleep, pain, and stress.

The study found that the patients who were grounded during sleep had reduced nighttime levels of cortisol and an overall normalization of cortisol secretion during the day. Remember, cortisol is the arch nemesis of sleep. If your cortisol levels are off, your sleep will be off. Subjective reporting by the study participants also indicated that grounding during sleep improved sleep quality, reduced pain, and lowered stress.

Getting yourself grounded can have a life-changing impact on your sleep quality. Now, I'm not implying that you need to go camping outside every night just to get all these benefits. Today you can utilize incredible earthing technology that brings the benefits of the earth's energy right into your home.

I've been using an earthing mat under my desk and sleeping on earthing sheets for about 7 years. These are well-designed products that can be connected to a grounding rod outside your home, or easily into the grounding plug you'll find in most electrical outlets. They safely and effectively deliver the free electrons from the earth right to you, and all you need to do is touch them with any part of your body. The above sleep study utilized grounding products to connect the test subjects with the earth, which triggered all of the impressive results they received.

I also had the opportunity to ask the incomparable Jeff Spencer, DC, about earthing with his patients. Dr. Spencer is an Olympic athlete and 8-time Tour de France–winning team doctor and has been directly involved in more than 40 Olympic, World, National, or Tour de France Championships. He told me that grounding technologies played a vital role in the success of his athletes. He found very quickly that earthing accelerated tissue repair and wound healing from injuries that athletes encountered during practice and competition. Among the benefits he also observed and reported from his patients: better sleep, less pain, more energy, and faster recovery.

The great news is that you don't have to be a world-class athlete to enjoy these types of benefits for yourself. Whether or not you decide to utilize these advancements in grounding technology, it's absolutely critical to get your body in contact with the earth on a regular basis to displace the positive charge you're carrying; to absorb free electrons to improve your recovery, heart health, and hormones; and, most important, to get a great night's sleep.

◇ ◇ ◇ ◇

GET GROUNDED
POWER TIP #1

Get your direct vitamin G. Make it a regular practice to get some quality time with your bare feet on the ground. This means conductive surfaces like soil, grass, sand (at the beach), and even living bodies of water like the ocean. There are other surfaces that are conductive, like concrete and brick, but their effectiveness depends on several factors. It's best to get your vitamin G (your daily interaction with the earth) from the soil and grass itself. By the way, have you ever noticed that when you take a vacation and go to a beach, you tend to get really amazing sleep? A lot of people actually fall asleep *at* the beach before they can even make it back inside. Now you know it's not a coincidence; it's the natural response of someone who finally gets connected with the earth again.

As for the amount of earthing time to target, Dr. Sinatra says, "Grounding to the earth changes your physiology immediately. The more you ground, the more you can benefit because you are at your most natural electrical state when connected to the earth." That said, even a minute is helpful, but the longer the better. I'd say to target a minimum of 10 minutes each day. And even if the allure of earthing isn't compelling enough for you yet, kicking off your shoes and stepping on the ground is great for strengthening your feet, improving your proprioception (how your brain can sense your body, as well as its position and movement through space), and improving your range of motion by increasing the flexibility and mobility of your feet. Being barefoot more often is a great overall health practice for many reasons.

GET GROUNDED
POWER TIP #2

If you live in a climate where getting your quality vitamin G time isn't always feasible, that's when access to earthing technology can be so helpful. The earthing products also allow you to not shift your life around too much to get the benefits of earthing. You can simply continue doing things you normally do—work at your computer, sleep, etc.—and be connected to the earth the whole time. You can have one earthing product or earthing products everywhere—there are mats, sheets, mattresses, mouse pads, and even bands you can put on specific pain points on your body that are used clinically to reduce pain and inflammation.

I was cautious of using the earthing sheets in the beginning because I was working to eliminate EMFs and to remove any unnecessary electronics from my bedroom. However, I was blown away to find that numerous studies, including one published in *European Biology and Bioelectromagnetics*, demonstrate that earthing immediately reduces the electric fields that are generated within the human body. Authors of the study found that "grounding essentially eliminates the ambient voltage induced on the body from common electricity power sources." Bottom line: Grounding can protect your cells from the issues associated with EMFs that we talked about in Chapter 12. Remember, nothing replaces getting in direct contact with the earth, but these items can be a great alternative to get the benefits you need. Check out the Sleep Smarter bonus resource guide for more information on these devices.

Because grounding has been proven to sync your body's circadian clock with the normal diurnal patterns of the earth, getting grounded after a flight is a smart thing to do. I've found that this practice virtually eliminates jet lag and helps me to adjust to a new time zone a lot faster. Humans were not designed to skip time zones in a few hours, so utilizing advances like this can really help to revitalize you. If at all possible, I get some direct vitamin G from the earth after travel. Plus, I bring my earthing sheets with me, and I always get a great night's sleep just like when I'm at home.

◇ ◇ ◇ ◇

The final tip is to have fun, experiment, and put the Sleep Smarter principles to work for you on a consistent basis. Stack the conditions in your favor to make great sleep an inevitable part of your life. It's not about being perfect, it's about making progress. And now it's time to put it all together for the greatest results possible, so let's dive right in to the 14-Day Sleep Makeover!

THE 14-DAY
SLEEP
MAKEOVER

Humans are creatures of habit and habitat. We've covered how to make your environment more sleep-friendly, how to put your body in the ideal *state* for sleep before bed, and even practices to calm your mind and put you in the mood for restful sleep. Now it's time to put these things together in a succinct pattern that really works for you long term.

Your brain loves to fall into patterns so that it can free up space to do other things. The more unconscious competencies we have, the more apt we are to have greater success and productivity.

What is an unconscious competency?

Well, there are ultimately four stages to learning any new skill or habit.

1. Unconscious incompetence—when you're doing something wrong and you don't know you're doing it wrong

2. Conscious incompetence—when you're doing something wrong and you know you're doing it wrong

3. Conscious competence—when you're doing something right but you have to consciously focus on doing it the right way

4. Unconscious competence—when you're doing something right and you don't even have to think about it

Initially, putting the things that you've learned in this book into action will place you in a phase of conscious competence. You're going to have to think about them and put conscious effort into doing them right. It's sort of like when you first learn to drive. You're very mindful of everything, and you have a checklist when you get into your car: First you might adjust the seat, then the mirrors, then your seat belt, etc., and you make sure you have them right before you start driving. While driving, you're hyperaware: eyes moving, paying attention to your speed, monitoring road signs and other cars, and being extra careful.

Then fast-forward a few months. When you hop in your car, the key goes in the ignition and you're out of there. You're not being reckless by any means, but you have the checklist automated. Your brain notices that the seat and mirrors are in the correct positions even without your conscious awareness needing to go there. The driving process itself can become so second nature that you can get into your car for a 20-minute drive and not even consciously remember all the steps you took to arrive at your destination.

It's not that you were hypnotized by an evil mutant; it's that your brain has freed up space to do other things because driving has become a strong unconscious competence. Your conscious mind can hop in if there's an irregularity or problem, but overall your brain has this activity on cruise control.

To get great sleep every night on cruise control, you simply need to ritualize things just like when you first learn to drive. The word *ritual* is derived from the Latin word *ritus*, meaning "a proven way of doing something." A ritual is a small sequence of step-by-step actions that put you in a certain mood, state, or frame of mind for getting something done.

Whether or not you've had a history of sleep problems, a regular bedtime ritual will help you wind down and prepare your body for the best sleep possible.

Jessica Alexander of the Sleep Council states, "A bedtime ritual teaches the brain to become familiar with sleep times and wake times. It programs the brain and internal body clock to get used to a set routine."

Parents throughout time are well aware of the power of bedtime rituals for their kids. Some of these rituals may include a warm bath, putting on pajamas, a bedtime story, relaxing music, or something as simple as a kiss on the forehead and a loving tuck into bed.

If you establish a consistent bedtime ritual, your kids drift off to sleep before you know it. Their brains and bodies have completely linked those systematic activities to going right to sleep. And, as I said before, in many ways we're just big adult babies, and the same basic programming is still there. We just need to learn to tap into it.

Lawrence Epstein, MD, instructor in medicine at Harvard Medical School, says, "Our body craves routine and likes to know what's coming." By creating a pre-sleep ritual, you're establishing a clear association between specific activities and your sleep.

Let's jump into the overview of your 14-Day Sleep Makeover to ensure you have the tools to get the best sleep ever.

THE GAME PLAN

As we discussed in Chapter 2, getting a great night's sleep starts the moment you wake up in the morning. Sleeping smarter and getting the best sleep of your life is set in place by having bedtime *and* daytime rituals. Each day of the 14-Day Sleep Makeover, we will be making small strides in both so that you can reach your desired destination with ease and grace.

You can begin the 14-Day Makeover anytime, but I recommend starting when you have a minimal amount of big distractions in your life. For example, if you are right in the middle of traveling for business, or working on a project due in a couple of days, great sleep is going to help tremendously, but you might want to postpone the full 14-day program until you have more control of your schedule. Whether you are starting tomorrow or in 2 weeks, the number one thing to do right now is to schedule your start date and completion date. Use your Outlook or Google calendar, or a physical calendar if you wish. All that matters is that you get it scheduled.

At no time during your sleep makeover should you feel overburdened or stressed. These strategies are here to make your life easier, not harder. They will generally require minimal time, and I want to remind you to be flexible and patient with yourself.

Each day will include some brief journal exercises that you can complete right here in this book or in your personal notebook or journal, or you can print out the PDF version found at sleepsmarterbook.com/bonus. These exercises are incredibly important because they will track your results. You may have heard the statement, "You can't manage what you can't measure," so it's very valuable to actually track your progress. Part of the journal exercises will be to give a Sleep Smarter Score that assesses where you are that day. Your scores are on a scale of 1 to 10, with 10 being the absolute best.

Review Sleep Makeover Day 1, then begin the following morning so that you'll know exactly what to do. Now that we've covered the game plan, let's dive right into your 14-Day Sleep Makeover!

Sleep Makeover Prep Day

Today is all about getting ready, which means taking inventory of where you are right now. Chances are you have already employed some of the strategies in this book because you were so excited to put them in play. So I want to give you a questionnaire to assess where you are right now *or* you can mark down where you started (if today isn't the first day you've been utilizing the Sleep Smarter strategies).

GETTING STARTED QUESTIONNAIRE

Answer the following questions on a scale of 1 to 10.

How would you rate your sleep right now?

|_____|

(1 = My sleep is a wreck   10 = My sleep is fantastic)

How do you feel physically when you get out of bed in the morning?

|_____|

(1 = Lots of pain   10 = No pain in sight)

How is your energy when you first get out of bed in the morning?

|_____|

(1 = Totally drained   10 = Totally refreshed and ready to take on the world!)

How do you feel mentally when you get out of bed in the morning?

|_____|

(1 = Foggy and agitated   10 = Optimistic and happy)

How consistent is your energy throughout the day?

|_____|

(1 = I can't keep myself awake all day   10 = I have great energy all day long)

Your official 14-Day Sleep Makeover starts tomorrow morning, so go ahead and review Day 1 so that you'll know exactly what to do. You're going to write in your journal two very quick times each day—10 to 15 minutes after you wake up, and 10 to 15 minutes before you go to bed each night. It's best to keep this book or your journal somewhere that you'll have easy access at both points in the day. Let's take a look and get ready for Day 1!

DAY 1

SLEEP MAKEOVER DAY 1 TARGETS

Morning: Time to set the tone for a great day and great sleep! After your standard morning rituals (using the bathroom, having some coffee or a couple glasses of water), now it's time to do a little exercise to get your heart rate up and encourage the secretion of natural "daytime hormones" to set your circadian rhythms on track. If you're not already a morning exerciser, then just start with 5 to 10 minutes of any of the following: bodyweight exercises (featured in the bonus resource guide at sleepsmarterbook.com/bonus), a brisk walk, rebounding on a mini-trampoline, Tabata, or a power yoga session.

Go ahead and get ready for your day now (shower, get dressed, or whatever you need to do), and then have breakfast. Breakfast will always follow the guidelines laid out in Chapter 13 to keep insulin down throughout the first part of the day to optimize hormone function and fat loss. Have your choice of protein, healthy fats, and nonstarchy veggies, or follow the sample plan in the bonus resource guide. Head into your day and have a great one.

Evening: Relaxation before bed is essential. You're going to discover that maintaining an evening ritual is like having an off switch for the stress in your life. We tend to get ready for everything else—we get ready for a date, we get ready for exercise or a sport, we get ready for work—but when it comes to sleep, many of us tend to just stumble into it or eventually pass out from exhaustion (and remember, there's a big difference between getting high-quality sleep and passing out!). So from now on you're going to treat getting ready for bed like getting ready for a hot date. You have a special indulgence you get to enjoy that's going to make you feel really *good* and will make everything in your life exponentially better. We're going to start getting ready for your date by closing the laptop, turning off the TV, and simply getting off any other electronic device that would compromise your quality time with your best friend, sleep. Get off of your devices at least 1 hour before your desired bedtime and do one of the following things:

- Read a book—preferably fiction. I used to think that reading fiction was unproductive, but now I realize that it's actually helped so many other areas in my life (from coming up with ideas to improving communication). It's not a surprise that kids sleep better than most adults. Reading fiction or having someone else read you fiction is powerful for relaxing our overused, analytical left brain. There are few things more capable of disconnecting you from your stress, worries, and tension than escaping to another world within the pages of a book.

  Nonfiction can be okay if it's a biography or something along those lines. But the best bet is to choose something other than the analytical, methodical, teaching, or training types of books. Ideally, you don't want to read anything that reminds you of work right before bed.

  Also, where you read may be important, too. Dr. Lawrence Epstein advises creating a clear association between your bed and sleep. It's recommended that you read anywhere in your home other than your bed itself if you don't have this strong association built. You can read in your bedroom, just not in your bed if you can't handle the reading rainbow juice.
- Listen to a podcast or audio book.
- Talk with a loved one: Significant other, kids, best friend—going over the day with someone you love, playing a board game, or talking about your plans for the future are some great things to do.
- Meditate.
- Journal—You'll need to fill out your Sleep Smarter Journal 10 to 15 minutes before bed, but we'll talk more about journaling on Day 2.
- Take a bath or shower.
- Any combination of the above.

After you choose an activity other than more screen time, the final thing on the agenda today is to fill out your daily journal entry.

DAY 1 JOURNAL

Fill out 10 to 15 minutes before going to bed.

On a scale of 1 to 10, rate your Overall Success Score for the day.
(How do you feel you did completing the Sleep Makeover assignments?)

|_____|

What was the best part of today's program?

_____

_____

_____

What was the toughest part (if any)?

_____

_____

_____

What do you feel you can improve on?

_____

_____

_____

What are you excited about for tomorrow?

_____

_____

_____

You'll start out by filling out your Overall Success Score tomorrow, so head to bed at your desired time, and that's all for today! I'll see you tomorrow to keep building on this momentum!

DAY 2

Fill out 10 to 15 minutes after getting up in the morning. Answer the following questions on a scale of 1 to 10.

How would you rate your sleep right now?

(1 = My sleep is a wreck   10 = My sleep is fantastic)

How do you feel physically when you get out of bed in the morning?

(1 = Lots of pain   10 = No pain in sight)

How is your energy when you first get out of bed in the morning?

(1 = Totally drained   10 = Totally refreshed and ready to take on the world!)

How do you feel mentally when you get out of bed in the morning?

(1 = Foggy and agitated   10 = Optimistic and happy)

How consistent is your energy throughout the day?

(1 = I can't keep myself awake all day   10 = I have great energy all day long)

SLEEP MAKEOVER DAY 2 TARGETS

Morning: After your standard morning rituals, hit 5 to 10 minutes of exercise just like yesterday. Afterward, get ready for your day, have breakfast, and head out.

Today's special assignment: Purchase or order some topical magnesium. We talked in depth about the importance of this in Chapter 7. Go back and review just how valuable magnesium can be to your sleep and health overall. The only topical magnesium I use, Ease Magnesium, is listed in the bonus resource guide, but there are many other options out there. Do this now so that you'll have it to use within the next couple days.

Evening: Continue getting ready for your sleep date. Shut off the screens 1 hour before your desired bedtime and do another chosen nighttime activity.

Tonight, take greater advantage of journaling. Of course you have the Sleep Makeover Journal, but you can go beyond that. This is a powerful practice that some of the most successful people in the world do. From Oprah to Tony Robbins, journaling has been a consistent part of their lives. For the intents of a pre-bedtime ritual, you can use your journal to capture stray thoughts and to get any of the random ideas out of your head and out onto the paper. That alone will help free up mental space. You could also use the journal as a check-in to look at your progress and affirm what steps you need to take next. Again, getting it out of your head and onto the paper can be very beneficial to achieving your goals.

A *gratitude log* or *gratitude journal* is another great idea. Part of the reason people have anxiety and trouble sleeping is a fixation on the things they haven't done and what they don't have. If you're reading this right now, chances are you are far more fortunate than you realize, and you may have gotten out of touch with just how much you have to be grateful for.

You can use a gratitude log to simply capture three to five things that you were grateful for today. They could be big things, or they could be small things (anything from seeing someone special smile to having great meals, to winning an award, to reaching an important milestone or anything else). Just the act of paying attention and writing them down to end your day will make you more receptive to all of the good things that happen that we end up taking for granted. In addition, research has shown that we have an increase in serotonin when we feel significant or important. Journaling and keeping a gratitude log can help you to remember and affirm the innate value you have and why you truly matter.

Jot down in the Day 2 Journal (or in the separate PDF journal) three things that you're grateful for today.

DAY 2 JOURNAL

Fill out 10 to 15 minutes before going to bed.

What are three things you're grateful for today?

1. _____

_____

_____

_____

_____

2. _____

_____

_____

_____

_____

3. _____

_____

_____

_____

_____

On a scale of 1 to 10, rate your Overall Success Score for the day.
(How do you feel you did completing the Sleep Makeover assignments?)

|_____|

What was the best part of today's program?

_____

_____

_____

_____

What was the toughest part (if any)?

_____

_____

_____

_____

What do you feel you can improve on?

_____

_____

_____

_____

What are you excited about for tomorrow?

_____

_____

_____

_____

DAY 3

SLEEP MAKEOVER DAY 3 QUESTIONNAIRE

Fill out 10 to 15 minutes after getting up in the morning. Answer the following questions on a scale of 1 to 10.

How would you rate your sleep right now?

|_____|

(1 = My sleep is a wreck   10 = My sleep is fantastic)

How do you feel physically when you get out of bed in the morning?

|_____|

(1 = Lots of pain   10 = No pain in sight)

How is your energy when you first get out of bed in the morning?

|_____|

(1 = Totally drained   10 = Totally refreshed and ready to take on the world!)

How do you feel mentally when you get out of bed in the morning?

|_____|

(1 = Foggy and agitated   10 = Optimistic and happy)

How consistent is your energy throughout the day?

|_____|

(1 = I can't keep myself awake all day   10 = I have great energy all day long)

SLEEP MAKEOVER DAY 3 TARGETS

Morning: After your standard morning rituals, hit 5 to 10 minutes of exercise just like yesterday. Today, focus on getting 10 minutes of direct sunlight as well. If this is during your exercise already, then that's great. If you haven't been seeing the sun very much, it's time to add it in! Weather permitting, you can do your exercise outside as mentioned, sit outside and do some daily reading, eat breakfast or lunch outside, or just relax outside getting some earthing in (which we'll talk more about soon). After pinning down when you'll get your sunlight in, get ready for your day, have breakfast, and head out.

Today's special assignment: From today forward, make sure that you finish any desired caffeine consumption before noon. As you know from Chapter 4, consuming caffeine even several hours before bedtime can interrupt your sleep. That stops today.

Also, today is about detoxing your bedroom and beginning to create your own sleep sanctuary. Get all unnecessary electronics out of your bedroom by following the recommendations in Chapter 12. TVs, laptops, smartphones, etc.—as the research shows, these things are disrupting the communication between the cells in your body, and they are definitely disturbing your sleep.

Evening: Continue getting ready for your sleep date. Shut off the screens 1 hour before your desired bedtime and do another chosen nighttime activity.

Right before bed, rub on the topical magnesium if you already have it. Use it liberally, following the recommendations in Chapter 7. Also, make sure to have a nice, cool temperature in your bedroom to facilitate deep sleep. Have the thermostat set so that it doesn't get any higher than 70°F (the ideal range is between 62° and 68°F, so the cooler the better).

DAY 3 JOURNAL

Fill out 10 to 15 minutes before going to bed.

What are three things you're grateful for today?

1. _____

_____

_____

_____

_____

2. _____

_____

_____

_____

_____

3. _____

_____

_____

_____

_____

On a scale of 1 to 10, rate your Overall Success Score for the day.
(How do you feel you did completing the Sleep Makeover assignments?)

|_____|

What was the best part of today's program?

_____

_____

_____

_____

What was the toughest part (if any)?

_____

_____

_____

_____

What do you feel you can improve on?

_____

_____

_____

_____

What are you excited about for tomorrow?

_____

_____

_____

_____

DAY 4

SLEEP MAKEOVER DAY 4 QUESTIONNAIRE

Fill out 10 to 15 minutes after getting up in the morning. Answer the following questions on a scale of 1 to 10.

How would you rate your sleep right now?

|_____|

(1 = My sleep is a wreck   10 = My sleep is fantastic)

How do you feel physically when you get out of bed in the morning?

|_____|

(1 = Lots of pain   10 = No pain in sight)

How is your energy when you first get out of bed in the morning?

|_____|

(1 = Totally drained   10 = Totally refreshed and ready to take on the world!)

How do you feel mentally when you get out of bed in the morning?

|_____|

(1 = Foggy and agitated   10 = Optimistic and happy)

How consistent is your energy throughout the day?

|_____|

(1 = I can't keep myself awake all day   10 = I have great energy all day long)

SLEEP MAKEOVER DAY 4 TARGETS

Morning: After your standard morning rituals, hit 5 to 10 minutes of exercise just like yesterday. Focus on getting 10 minutes of direct sunlight today as well. Get ready for your day, have breakfast, and head out.

Today's special assignment: Time to continue creating your own sleep sanctuary. Hop online or head to the store and purchase some blackout curtains for your bedroom. Also, get yourself one of the recommended plants that can aid in your air quality and sleep quality, as mentioned in Chapter 8. You can find resources for all of these in the bonus resource guide.

Evening: Continue getting ready for your sleep date. Shut off the screens 1 hour before your desired bedtime and do another chosen nighttime activity.

Make sure your blackout curtains are set up and your plant is by your bedside (if these are on their way via mail, that's okay; you'll have them soon enough!). Right before bed, rub on the topical magnesium if you already have it. Be sure to have a nice, cool temperature in your bedroom to facilitate deep sleep.

DAY 4 JOURNAL

Fill out 10 to 15 minutes before going to bed.

What are three things you're grateful for today?

1. _____

_____

_____

_____

_____

2. _____

_____

_____

_____

_____

3. _____

_____

_____

_____

_____

On a scale of 1 to 10, rate your Overall Success Score for the day.
(How do you feel you did completing the Sleep Makeover assignments?)

| |

What was the best part of today's program?

_____

_____

_____

_____

What was the toughest part (if any)?

_____

_____

_____

_____

What do you feel you can improve on?

_____

_____

_____

_____

What are you excited about for tomorrow?

_____

_____

_____

_____

DAY 5

SLEEP MAKEOVER DAY 5 QUESTIONNAIRE

Fill out 10 to 15 minutes after getting up in the morning. Answer the following questions on a scale of 1 to 10.

How would you rate your sleep right now?

|_____|

(1 = My sleep is a wreck   10 = My sleep is fantastic)

How do you feel physically when you get out of bed in the morning?

|_____|

(1 = Lots of pain   10 = No pain in sight)

How is your energy when you first get out of bed in the morning?

|_____|

(1 = Totally drained   10 = Totally refreshed and ready to take on the world!)

How do you feel mentally when you get out of bed in the morning?

|_____|

(1 = Foggy and agitated   10 = Optimistic and happy)

How consistent is your energy throughout the day?

|_____|

(1 = I can't keep myself awake all day   10 = I have great energy all day long)

SLEEP MAKEOVER DAY 5 TARGETS

Morning: After your standard morning rituals, it's time to add in a new, valuable component of your Sleep Smarter plan. Add in 5 to 10 minutes of meditation (aka brain training) using a practice you already have or one of the resources in the bonus resource guide. There are great apps you can use, guided meditations, and more to help take your energy, focus, and health to the next level. After meditation, hit 5 to 10 minutes of exercise. Focus on getting 10 minutes of direct sunlight today as well. Get ready for your day, have breakfast, and head out.

Today's special assignment: Book a massage for yourself this week. We talked in depth about the benefits in Chapter 19. If a massage is not in your budget right now, make a date with a friend or significant other to exchange massages. It will be a fun—and relaxing—way to catch up, and it'll benefit your health as well. You deserve it!

Evening: Get ready for your sleep date. Shut off the screens *90 minutes* before your desired bedtime and do another chosen nighttime activity.

Right before bed, rub on the topical magnesium. Make sure to have a nice, cool temperature in your bedroom to facilitate deep sleep.

DAY 5 JOURNAL

Fill out 10 to 15 minutes before going to bed.

What are three things you're grateful for today?

1. _____

_____

_____

_____

_____

2. _____

_____

_____

_____

_____

3. _____

_____

_____

On a scale of 1 to 10, rate your Overall Success Score for the day.
(How do you feel you did completing the Sleep Makeover assignments?)

|_____|

What was the best part of today's program?

_____
_____
_____
_____

What was the toughest part (if any)?

_____
_____
_____
_____

What do you feel you can improve on?

_____
_____
_____
_____

What are you excited about for tomorrow?

_____
_____
_____
_____

DAY 6

SLEEP MAKEOVER DAY 6 QUESTIONNAIRE

Fill out 10 to 15 minutes after getting up in the morning. Answer the following questions on a scale of 1 to 10.

How would you rate your sleep right now?

|_____|

(1 = My sleep is a wreck   10 = My sleep is fantastic)

How do you feel physically when you get out of bed in the morning?

|_____|

(1 = Lots of pain   10 = No pain in sight)

How is your energy when you first get out of bed in the morning?

|_____|

(1 = Totally drained   10 = Totally refreshed and ready to take on the world!)

How do you feel mentally when you get out of bed in the morning?

|_____|

(1 = Foggy and agitated   10 = Optimistic and happy)

How consistent is your energy throughout the day?

|_____|

(1 = I can't keep myself awake all day   10 = I have great energy all day long)

SLEEP MAKEOVER DAY 6 TARGETS

Morning: After your standard morning rituals, score 5 to 10 minutes of meditation (aka brain training). After meditation, hit 5 to 10 minutes of exercise. Focus on getting 10 minutes of direct sunlight today as well. Get ready for your day, have breakfast, and head out.

Today's special assignment: Focus on optimizing the time you go to sleep and the time you wake up. As you know from Chapter 6, the most valuable hormone production, enzymatic repair, and more is achieved by getting sleep between the hours of 10:00 p.m. and 2:00 a.m. Again, this has variance based on the time of year and other factors, but shoot for getting as much of this "money time" as possible. Hopefully you've been employing the gradual method of moving your bedtime and wake time up by 15-minute increments covered in Chapter 18. If you haven't, now is the time to do so. If you're not at your desired bedtime yet, move your bedtime up by 15 minutes every other day until you hit your goal. For example, if your desired bedtime is 10:30 p.m. and you've been getting to bed at 11:30 p.m., ensure that you are in bed by 11:15 p.m. tonight. Continue to build and move gracefully from there. Correspondingly, move your wake time up 15 minutes earlier as well if you've had a habit of staying in bed late. Just ensure that you are getting the target number of hours of sleep that you feel great about.

Evening: Get ready for your sleep date. Shut off the screens *90 minutes* before your desired bedtime and do another chosen nighttime activity.

Right before bed, rub on the topical magnesium. Make sure to have a nice, cool temperature in your bedroom to facilitate deep sleep.

DAY 6 JOURNAL

Fill out 10 to 15 minutes before going to bed.

What are three things you're grateful for today?

1. _____

_____

_____

_____

_____

2. _____

_____

_____

_____

_____

3. _____

_____

_____

_____

_____

On a scale of 1 to 10, rate your Overall Success Score for the day.
(How do you feel you did completing the Sleep Makeover assignments?)

|_____|

What was the best part of today's program?

_____

_____

_____

_____

What was the toughest part (if any)?

_____

_____

_____

_____

What do you feel you can improve on?

_____

_____

_____

_____

What are you excited about for tomorrow?

_____

_____

_____

_____

DAY 7

SLEEP MAKEOVER DAY 7 QUESTIONNAIRE

Fill out 10 to 15 minutes after getting up in the morning. Answer the following questions on a scale of 1 to 10.

How would you rate your sleep right now?

|_____|

(1 = My sleep is a wreck   10 = My sleep is fantastic)

How do you feel physically when you get out of bed in the morning?

|_____|

(1 = Lots of pain   10 = No pain in sight)

How is your energy when you first get out of bed in the morning?

|_____|

(1 = Totally drained   10 = Totally refreshed and ready to take on the world!)

How do you feel mentally when you get out of bed in the morning?

|_____|

(1 = Foggy and agitated   10 = Optimistic and happy)

How consistent is your energy throughout the day?

|_____|

(1 = I can't keep myself awake all day   10 = I have great energy all day long)

SLEEP MAKEOVER DAY 7 TARGETS

Morning: After your standard morning rituals, score 5 to 10 minutes of meditation (aka brain training). After meditation, hit 5 *to* 15 minutes of exercise. Focus on getting 10 minutes of direct sunlight today as well. Get ready for your day, have breakfast, and head out.

Today's special assignment: Simply add in 5 to 10 minutes more of morning exercise and/or meditation from today forward since you are now getting up a bit earlier to take advantage of the day.

Evening: Get ready for your sleep date. Shut off the screens 90 minutes before your desired bedtime and do another chosen nighttime activity.

Right before bed, rub on the topical magnesium. Make sure to have a nice, cool temperature in your bedroom to facilitate deep sleep.

DAY 7 JOURNAL

Fill out 10 to 15 minutes before going to bed.

What are three things you're grateful for today?

1. _____

_____

_____

_____

_____

2. _____

_____

_____

_____

_____

3. _____

_____

_____

_____

_____

On a scale of 1 to 10, rate your Overall Success Score for the day.
(How do you feel you did completing the Sleep Makeover assignments?)

|_____|

What was the best part of today's program?

_____
_____
_____
_____

What was the toughest part (if any)?

_____
_____
_____
_____

What do you feel you can improve on?

_____
_____
_____
_____

What are you excited about for tomorrow?

_____
_____
_____
_____

DAY 8

SLEEP MAKEOVER DAY 8 QUESTIONNAIRE

Fill out 10 to 15 minutes after getting up in the morning. Answer the following questions on a scale of 1 to 10.

How would you rate your sleep right now?

(1 = My sleep is a wreck   10 = My sleep is fantastic)

How do you feel physically when you get out of bed in the morning?

(1 = Lots of pain   10 = No pain in sight)

How is your energy when you first get out of bed in the morning?

(1 = Totally drained   10 = Totally refreshed and ready to take on the world!)

How do you feel mentally when you get out of bed in the morning?

(1 = Foggy and agitated   10 = Optimistic and happy)

How consistent is your energy throughout the day?

(1 = I can't keep myself awake all day   10 = I have great energy all day long)

SLEEP MAKEOVER DAY 8 TARGETS

Morning: After your standard morning rituals, score 5 to 10 minutes of meditation (aka brain training). After meditation, hit 5 to 15 minutes of exercise. Focus on getting 10 minutes of direct sunlight today as well.

Get ready for your day, have breakfast, and head out.

Today's special assignment: Now that we are at the halfway mark, it's time to really shift our focus toward our food! As you learned in Chapter 7 and Chapter 13, the food we eat has a *huge* impact on our sleep and health overall. Starting today and moving forward, it's important to eat real, nutritious food at every meal and not just breakfast time. Be sure to get in at least five servings of the foods that contain the good-sleep nutrients discussed in Chapter 7 today, and each day moving forward. If you need more support on this, make sure to take advantage of the sample meal plan and more in the bonus resource guide. Not only are you going to sleep better, but you're going to optimize your hormones, lose body fat, and radically improve your energy levels.

Evening: Get ready for your sleep date. Shut off the screens 90 minutes before your desired bedtime and do another chosen nighttime activity.

Right before bed, rub on the topical magnesium. Make sure to have a nice, cool temperature in your bedroom to facilitate deep sleep.

DAY 8 JOURNAL

Fill out 10 to 15 minutes before going to bed.

What are three things you're grateful for today?

1. _____

_____

_____

_____

_____

2. _____

_____

_____

_____

_____

3. _____
_____
_____
_____
_____

On a scale of 1 to 10, rate your Overall Success Score for the day.
(How do you feel you did completing the Sleep Makeover assignments?)

|_____|

What was the best part of today's program?

_____
_____
_____
_____

What was the toughest part (if any)?

_____
_____
_____
_____

What do you feel you can improve on?

_____
_____
_____
_____

What are you excited about for tomorrow?

_____
_____
_____
_____

DAY 9

SLEEP MAKEOVER DAY 9 QUESTIONNAIRE

Fill out 10 to 15 minutes after getting up in the morning. Answer the following questions on a scale of 1 to 10.

How would you rate your sleep right now?

|_____|

(1 = My sleep is a wreck   10 = My sleep is fantastic)

How do you feel physically when you get out of bed in the morning?

|_____|

(1 = Lots of pain   10 = No pain in sight)

How is your energy when you first get out of bed in the morning?

|_____|

(1 = Totally drained   10 = Totally refreshed and ready to take on the world!)

How do you feel mentally when you get out of bed in the morning?

|_____|

(1 = Foggy and agitated   10 = Optimistic and happy)

How consistent is your energy throughout the day?

|_____|

(1 = I can't keep myself awake all day   10 = I have great energy all day long)

SLEEP MAKEOVER DAY 9 TARGETS

Morning: After your standard morning rituals, score 5 to 10 minutes of meditation (aka brain training). After meditation, hit 5 to 15 minutes of exercise. Focus on getting 10 minutes of direct sunlight today as well.

Get ready for your day, have breakfast, and head out.

Today's special assignment: Time to begin adding the final pieces to your sleep sanctuary. Get yourself some alternative lighting for your bedroom at night. It could be low-blue lightbulbs, it could be a salt lamp, it could be a lamp with a dimmer, or it could even be as simple (and timeless) as candles. For the environment outside of your bedroom, and what you can use as soon as the sun goes down to optimize melatonin production, get yourself some glasses that block blue light. And make sure that you've downloaded the blue light blocking apps to your devices for nighttime usage (especially when extenuating circumstances hit and you have to be on your devices later than normal). You can find access to all of these things and more in the resource guide.

Evening: Get ready for your sleep date. Shut off the screens 90 minutes before your desired bedtime and do another chosen nighttime activity. Utilize blue light blocking glasses as well as low-blue lightbulbs, or simply dim the lights if possible.

Right before bed, rub on the topical magnesium. Make sure to have a nice, cool temperature in your bedroom to facilitate deep sleep.

DAY 9 JOURNAL

Fill out 10 to 15 minutes before going to bed.

What are three things you're grateful for today?

1. _____

_____

_____

_____

_____

2. _____

_____

_____

_____

_____

3. _____

_____

_____

_____

_____

On a scale of 1 to 10, rate your Overall Success Score for the day.
(How do you feel you did completing the Sleep Makeover assignments?)

|_____|

What was the best part of today's program?

_____

_____

_____

_____

What was the toughest part (if any)?

_____

_____

_____

_____

What do you feel you can improve on?

_____

_____

_____

_____

What are you excited about for tomorrow?

_____

_____

_____

_____

Day 10

SLEEP MAKEOVER DAY 10 QUESTIONNAIRE

Fill out 10 to 15 minutes after getting up in the morning. Answer the following questions on a scale of 1 to 10.

How would you rate your sleep right now?

|_____|

(1 = My sleep is a wreck   10 = My sleep is fantastic)

How do you feel physically when you get out of bed in the morning?

|_____|

(1 = Lots of pain   10 = No pain in sight)

How is your energy when you first get out of bed in the morning?

|_____|

(1 = Totally drained   10 = Totally refreshed and ready to take on the world!)

How do you feel mentally when you get out of bed in the morning?

|_____|

(1 = Foggy and agitated   10 = Optimistic and happy)

How consistent is your energy throughout the day?

|_____|

(1 = I can't keep myself awake all day   10 = I have great energy all day long)

SLEEP MAKEOVER DAY 10 TARGETS

Morning: After your standard morning rituals, score 10 minutes of meditation (aka brain training). After meditation, hit 5 to 15 minutes of exercise. Focus on getting 10 minutes of direct sunlight today as well. Get ready for your day, have breakfast, and head out.

Today's special assignment: Getting yourself grounded can be a game changer. No, I'm not talking about when you got in trouble as a kid (I don't even want to know what you did to get grounded)—I'm talking about getting yourself connected to the diurnal patterns and free electrons of the earth that we covered in Chapter 21. Today and moving forward, add in at least 10 minutes of earthing each day.

You can do many of the activities mentioned in this book while getting your earth on. Exercise, meditation (qigong and tai chi are excellent to do while earthing), reading, soaking up the sun, having a meal, and many other things you're already doing can be done while having your bare feet in contact with the earth. You can also opt to get yourself some earthing bed sheets and/or an earthing office mat for your desk. I love the earthing technology so much that it's one of my favorite gifts to give to the people I care about. It's not a must if you're already getting in some earthing time each day, but it sure does make getting the benefits we went over in Chapter 21 a lot more convenient. You can get much more information on earthing and earthing products in the bonus resource guide.

Evening: Get ready for your sleep date. Shut off the screens 90 minutes before your desired bedtime and do another chosen nighttime activity. Utilize blue light blocking glasses as well as low-blue lightbulbs, or simply dim the lights if possible.

Right before bed, rub on the topical magnesium. Make sure to have a nice, cool temperature in your bedroom to facilitate deep sleep.

DAY 10 JOURNAL

Fill out 10 to 15 minutes before going to bed.

What are three things you're grateful for today?

1. _____

_____

_____

_____

_____

2. _____

_____

_____

_____

_____

3. _____

_____

_____

_____

_____

On a scale of 1 to 10, rate your Overall Success Score for the day.
(How do you feel you did completing the Sleep Makeover assignments?)

|_____|

What was the best part of today's program?

_____

_____

_____

_____

What was the toughest part (if any)?

_____

_____

_____

_____

What do you feel you can improve on?

_____

_____

_____

_____

What are you excited about for tomorrow?

_____

_____

_____

_____

DAY 11

Fill out 10 to 15 minutes after getting up in the morning. Answer the following questions on a scale of 1 to 10.

How would you rate your sleep right now?

(1 = My sleep is a wreck   10 = My sleep is fantastic)

How do you feel physically when you get out of bed in the morning?

(1 = Lots of pain   10 = No pain in sight)

How is your energy when you first get out of bed in the morning?

(1 = Totally drained   10 = Totally refreshed and ready to take on the world!)

How do you feel mentally when you get out of bed in the morning?

(1 = Foggy and agitated   10 = Optimistic and happy)

How consistent is your energy throughout the day?

(1 = I can't keep myself awake all day   10 = I have great energy all day long)

SLEEP MAKEOVER DAY 11 TARGETS

Morning: After your standard morning rituals, score 10 minutes of meditation (aka brain training). After meditation, hit 5 to 15 minutes of exercise. Focus on getting 10 minutes of direct sunlight today as well. Get ready for your day, have breakfast, and head out.

Today's special assignment: In Chapter 20 we talked in depth about how much the clothes we wear affect our health. Today, make it a mandate to lose the restrictive, tight-fitting clothes at least while you sleep. This is a very simple fix, so just put it in play from this day forward.

Evening: Get ready for your sleep date. Shut off the screens 90 minutes before your desired bedtime and do another chosen nighttime activity. Utilize blue light blocking glasses as well as low-blue lightbulbs, or simply dim the lights if possible.

Right before bed, rub on the topical magnesium. Make sure to have a nice, cool temperature in your bedroom to facilitate deep sleep.

DAY 11 JOURNAL

Fill out 10 to 15 minutes before going to bed.

What are three things you're grateful for today?

1. _____

_____

_____

_____

_____

2. _____

_____

_____

_____

_____

3. _____

_____

_____

_____

_____

On a scale of 1 to 10, rate your Overall Success Score for the day.
(How do you feel you did completing the Sleep Makeover assignments?)

| |

What was the best part of today's program?

_____

_____

_____

_____

What was the toughest part (if any)?

_____

_____

_____

_____

What do you feel you can improve on?

_____

_____

_____

_____

What are you excited about for tomorrow?

_____

_____

_____

_____

DAY 12

SLEEP MAKEOVER DAY 12 QUESTIONNAIRE

Fill out 10 to 15 minutes after getting up in the morning. Answer the following questions on a scale of 1 to 10.

How would you rate your sleep right now?

(1 = My sleep is a wreck   10 = My sleep is fantastic)

How do you feel physically when you get out of bed in the morning?

(1 = Lots of pain   10 = No pain in sight)

How is your energy when you first get out of bed in the morning?

(1 = Totally drained   10 = Totally refreshed and ready to take on the world!)

How do you feel mentally when you get out of bed in the morning?

(1 = Foggy and agitated   10 = Optimistic and happy)

How consistent is your energy throughout the day?

(1 = I can't keep myself awake all day   10 = I have great energy all day long)

SLEEP MAKEOVER DAY 12 TARGETS

Morning: After your standard morning rituals, score 10 minutes of meditation (aka brain training). After meditation, hit 5 to 15 minutes of exercise. Focus on getting 10 minutes of direct sunlight today as well. Get ready for your day, have breakfast, and head out.

Today's special assignment: Before bed this evening, as part of your nightly ritual, add in a little self-massage or other bodywork to help switch off the sympathetic nervous system (fight or flight) and switch *on* the parasympathetic nervous system (rest and digest). In Chapter 19 we went over some great strategies that you can employ. Review that chapter and take action on it tonight.

Evening: Get ready for your sleep date. Shut off the screens 90 minutes before your desired bedtime and do another chosen nighttime activity. Utilize blue light blocking glasses as well as low-blue lightbulbs, or simply dim the lights if possible.

Shortly before bed, devote 5 minutes to doing some bodywork or ask a loved one to give you a massage. Right before bed, rub on the topical magnesium. Make sure to have a nice, cool temperature in your bedroom to facilitate deep sleep.

DAY 12 JOURNAL

Fill out 10 to 15 minutes before going to bed.

What are three things you're grateful for today?

1. _____

_____

_____

_____

_____

2. _____

_____

_____

_____

_____

3. _____

_____

_____

_____

_____

On a scale of 1 to 10, rate your Overall Success Score for the day.
(How do you feel you did completing the Sleep Makeover assignments?)

|_____|

What was the best part of today's program?

_____

_____

_____

_____

What was the toughest part (if any)?

_____

_____

_____

_____

What do you feel you can improve on?

_____

_____

_____

_____

What are you excited about for tomorrow?

_____

_____

_____

_____

Day 13

SLEEP MAKEOVER DAY 13 QUESTIONNAIRE

Fill out 10 to 15 minutes after getting up in the morning. Answer the following questions on a scale of 1 to 10.

How would you rate your sleep right now?

(1 = My sleep is a wreck   10 = My sleep is fantastic)

How do you feel physically when you get out of bed in the morning?

(1 = Lots of pain   10 = No pain in sight)

How is your energy when you first get out of bed in the morning?

(1 = Totally drained   10 = Totally refreshed and ready to take on the world!)

How do you feel mentally when you get out of bed in the morning?

(1 = Foggy and agitated   10 = Optimistic and happy)

How consistent is your energy throughout the day?

(1 = I can't keep myself awake all day   10 = I have great energy all day long)

SLEEP MAKEOVER DAY 13 TARGETS

Morning: After your standard morning rituals, score 10 minutes of meditation (aka brain training). After meditation, hit 5 to 15 minutes of exercise. Focus on getting 10 minutes of direct sunlight today as well. Get ready for your day, have breakfast, and head out.

Today's special assignment: If you've been successful at utilizing the strategies thus far in the 14-Day Sleep Makeover but feel that you could still use a little bit more assistance at optimizing your sleep, then today is the day to add in some smart supplementation. Take advantage of any of the supplements we covered in Chapter 17, and check out the bonus resource guide for the best sources.

Evening: Get ready for your sleep date. Shut off the screens 90 minutes before your desired bedtime and do another chosen nighttime activity. Utilize blue light blocking glasses as well as low-blue lightbulbs, or simply dim the lights if possible.

Shortly before bed, devote 5 minutes to doing some bodywork or ask a loved one to give you a massage. Right before bed, rub on the topical magnesium. Make sure to have a nice, cool temperature in your bedroom to facilitate deep sleep.

DAY 13 JOURNAL

Fill out 10 to 15 minutes before going to bed.

What are three things you're grateful for today?

1. _____

_____

_____

_____

_____

2. _____

_____

_____

_____

_____

3. _____

_____

_____

_____

_____

On a scale of 1 to 10, rate your Overall Success Score for the day.
(How do you feel you did completing the Sleep Makeover assignments?)

| |

What was the best part of today's program?

_____

_____

_____

_____

What was the toughest part (if any)?

_____

_____

_____

_____

What do you feel you can improve on?

_____

_____

_____

_____

What are you excited about for tomorrow?

_____

_____

_____

_____

DAY 14

SLEEP MAKEOVER DAY 14 QUESTIONNAIRE

Fill out 10 to 15 minutes after getting up in the morning. Answer the following questions on a scale of 1 to 10.

How would you rate your sleep right now?

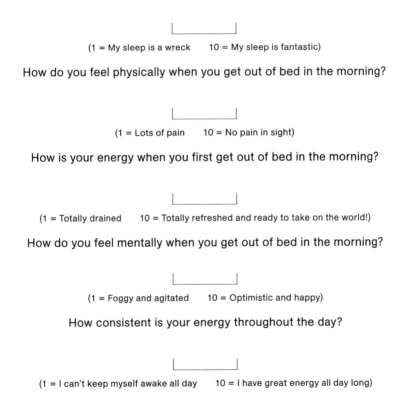

(1 = My sleep is a wreck   10 = My sleep is fantastic)

How do you feel physically when you get out of bed in the morning?

(1 = Lots of pain   10 = No pain in sight)

How is your energy when you first get out of bed in the morning?

(1 = Totally drained   10 = Totally refreshed and ready to take on the world!)

How do you feel mentally when you get out of bed in the morning?

(1 = Foggy and agitated   10 = Optimistic and happy)

How consistent is your energy throughout the day?

(1 = I can't keep myself awake all day   10 = I have great energy all day long)

SLEEP MAKEOVER DAY 14 TARGETS

Morning: After your standard morning rituals, score 10 minutes of meditation (aka brain training). After meditation, hit 5 to 15 minutes of exercise. Focus on getting 10 minutes of direct sunlight today as well.

Get ready for your day, have breakfast, and head out.

Today's special assignment: Optimize! Continue to build on the results you've already achieved. Be consistent, keep moving forward, and continue to put a priority on your health!

Evening: Get ready for your sleep date. Shut off the screens 90 minutes before your desired bedtime and do another chosen nighttime activity. Utilize blue light blocking glasses as well as low-blue lightbulbs, or simply dim the lights if possible.

Shortly before bed, devote 5 minutes to doing some bodywork or ask a loved one to give you a massage. Right before bed, rub on the topical magnesium. Make sure to have a nice, cool temperature in your bedroom to facilitate deep sleep.

DAY 14 JOURNAL

Fill out 10 to 15 minutes before going to bed.

What are three things you're grateful for today?

1. _____

_____

_____

_____

_____

2. _____

_____

_____

_____

_____

3. _____

_____

_____

On a scale of 1 to 10, rate your Overall Success Score for the day.
(How do you feel you did completing the Sleep Makeover assignments?)

|_____|

What was the best part of today's program?

_____

_____

_____

_____

What was the toughest part (if any)?

_____

_____

_____

_____

What do you feel you can improve on?

_____

_____

_____

_____

What are you excited about for tomorrow?

_____

_____

_____

_____

CONGRATULATIONS!

By completing this 14-Day Sleep Makeover, you have effectively upgraded the function of your hormones, improved your genetic expression, and created a solid foundation for the future. It's not what you do sometimes, but what you do consistently, that tells the real story of your results.

A wonderful quote from Samuel Johnson states, "The chains of habit are too small to be felt until they are too strong to be broken." Many of these habit changes may seem small in retrospect, but you are working to literally make them a part of who you are. By choosing to sleep smarter and put these strategies in place on a consistent basis, you are stacking so many conditions in your favor that it will make getting great results inevitable.

It's Time to Say Goodnight

Sleep is the secret sauce.

The human body is brilliantly designed to utilize sleep to improve virtually every function that you have. You don't plug into a socket. You are made anew by honoring your body and getting the sleep you require.

The path to success will not be made by bypassing dreamland. You require sleep to be the greatest version of yourself, and no pill, potion, or tactic can change that.

To be great at something, you have to make a study of it. I'm truly honored and happy that you picked up this book and decided to make a study of something that will bring you great health and happiness for many years to come.

In our world today, it's the simple things that help us reconnect with what is most valuable. It is my hope that this book helps you to reconnect with nature, reconnect with joy, and reconnect with what's most important about yourself.

ACKNOWLEDGMENTS

I feel that we are all patchwork quilts of the experiences and interactions that we've had in our lives. I know that I wouldn't be who I am or where I am without all of the incredible people who've impacted my life in one way or another. For that, I am eternally grateful.

First of all, I want to thank my wife, Anne. Without you, I'd be just a shell of who I am. You've taught me so much, you've made me better in every way, and you've trusted me more than anyone when I had these hare-brained ideas to change the world in a positive way. Thank you for loving me like you do. I will spend the rest of my life making yours as beautiful as possible. You deserve it!

I want to thank my kids: Braden, Jorden, and Jasné. You are my unyielding motivation. I am driven to be great because of you, for you. Braden, you are still a little guy when this book is released, but I want you to know that I have never smiled so much and laughed so much and been as happy since the day that you arrived in my life. I love you beyond words. Jorden, wow, you are such an incredible human being. Your attitude about life, the way you care about other people, how you are driven to be your very best. You inspire me so much, son! I really hope that you know that. Jasné, no matter how many years go by, you will still always be my baby girl. When you came along, it was the catalyst for me to step my game up. I had to figure out how to be a better father, a better teacher, and a better man because of you. I'm so proud of you, and I can't wait to see you achieve your dreams.

We all need encouragement, and we all need to feel like we matter. I want to give a special thank you to my middle-school English teacher Kathy Blackmore for praising me and encouraging me to write. You have no idea how much it meant to me when you published a piece of my writing in the school newspaper. I felt like I had value and that my words mattered. I needed that at that exact moment. I'm forever grateful for you.

During those formative years, no one was closer to me than my brother and sister. Darrell, thank you for being the other set of eyes to witness our life growing up. And thank you for being the other heart to experience it all with me. No one knows our story more than you do. I'm so proud of the man you are today. Your happiness is, and always will be, contagious, so keep on smiling, brother! Michelle, it's funny, you were so little while I was really growing into adulthood. I wish that I could have spent more time with you when we were all under the same roof. I think you are absolutely beautiful, inside and out. Keep moving forward, little sister. The best is yet to come!

A very special thank you to my mother and father. Thank you two for taking care of us the best way that you knew how. I know that you sacrificed so much, and I wouldn't have the courage, hustle, and strength that I have without you. Please take these years and live happier and fuller than you ever have. It's about time for that!

Without question, my most influential teacher in understand the greater design of health and wellness is my mother-in-law, Wambui. You are the most generous, inspiring, and enlightened person that I've ever met. I don't know where I'd be without your influence. Please know that every person I impact in a positive way is a direct result of the guidance from your hand. Thank you for believing in me.

It's also important to have a reference point to what's possible. Aunt Caroline, your audacity to go to college and to write really shifted my paradigm and gave me an example of what was possible for me. Proximity can be everything for a child (and as an adult for that matter!), and having you in my life inspired me more than you know.

The drive to write this book is really the result of two tremendously impactful things: working in my clinical practice, and devoting countless hours to creating my show. I want to thank every single one of my clients over the years. Thank you so much for trusting in me and having the courage to take action to improve your health. I want to think *ALL* of the listeners of *The Model Health Show!* We made this book a reality together. Thank you for making me a part of your life and for making a space for me to be the best teacher and motivator possible. Please know that much, much more greatness is in store!

My show wouldn't be possible without my incredible cohost and producer, Jade Harrell. You are a gift in my life and a gift in everyone's life who's fortunate enough to know you. I'm blown away every time I think of the reach and impact we've made. Thank you from the bottom of my heart for sharing your talents to help make this mission a reality.

Other members of *The Model Health Show* team—Bill "Shoe" Smith, Phil Crawford, Brett Oliver, Henk Jordaan, and Alpha Llanderal—thank you all so much for your contributions. You have helped to improve the lives of so many people. Let's keep taking it to the next level!

I want to thank all of the amazing guests who've graced *The Model Health Show* and help make it what it is. This list of superstars is growing, but please know that no one shines brighter than you! Catherine Garceau, Jonathan Bailor, Sean Croxton, Dr. Jennifer Hanes, Stacy Toth, Tristan Truscott, Sydney Ross Singer, Ty Bollinger, Daniel Vitalis, Dr. Pedram Shojai, Peter Ragnar, Abel James, Ty Bollinger, Jim Kwik, John Lee Dumas, Sarah Fragoso, Sheleana Jennings, Ameer Rosic, Jordan Harbinger, Pat Flynn, Dr. Sara Gottfried, Vinnie Tortorich, Dr. Kelly Starrett, Madelyn Moon, Travis Brewer, Evan Brand, Jimmy Moore, Prince Ea, Rae Mohrmann, Dr. William Davis, Jackie Joyner-Kersee, Rich Roll, Hal Elrod, Gretchen Rubin, Chalene Johnson, Alex Jamieson, Jairek Robbins, Ian Clark, Drew Manning, Bob Proctor, Steve Cook, Jeff Blake, Dr. Jeff Spencer, Eric "ET" Thomas, George Bryant, Katy Bowman, Lewis Howes, Steph Gaudreau, Mike Dolce, Dr. Jillian Teta, Ben Greenfield, Gunnar Lovelace, Darren and Danielle Natoni, thank you!

This book would not be possible without the amazing team at Rodale who has helped to put this project of change together. Marisa, Gail, Yelena, Izzy, Rachel, Emily, Sindy, Melissa, Karen, and the rest of the team, thank you all so much for contributing your time and talents to this. The strength, exuberance, positive energy, and skill that all of you have just blows me away. I instantly felt right at home with you, and I'm unbelievably honored to work with you.

My agents, Scott Hoffman and Steve Troha, what can I say? You two are the best in the business. Thank you for seeing my vision and helping to make it a reality. I'm forever grateful for having you in my life.

There are some special friends that I have to take a moment to thank for believing in me, inspiring me, and being a part of my story. Larry Hagner, Jim Kwik, Aubrey Marcus, George Bryant, Drew Manning, June Tate, Akhila Balaram, Ken and Susan Balk, Larry and Oksana Ostrovsky, Lori Dowd, and John Lee Dumas, thank you! And I want to give a special big thank you to the team at Onnit and the team at Thrive Market for the difference you're making on the planet!

There are so many other people that have had a positive impact on my life, the likes of which (and my gratitude for them) would take up another book itself. So, I want to close by saying, if we've ever shared a single moment together, thank you. Thank you for being a part of my story, and thank you for allowing me to be a part of yours.

REFERENCES

INTRODUCTION

Atlanta Snoring Institute. "Atlanta Snoring Institute Honors National Sleep Awareness Week by Providing Breakthrough Treatments and Cures." www.prweb.com/releases/pillar-procedure/atlanta/prweb 11643960.htm.

Division of Sleep Medicine at Harvard Medical School. "Mood and Sleep." http://healthysleep.med.harvard .edu/need-sleep/whats-in-it-for-you/mood.

Jean-Philippe Chaput, PhD, and Angelo Tremblay, PhD. "Adequate sleep to improve the treatment of obesity." *Canadian Medical Association Journal.* www.cmaj.ca/content/early/2012/09/17/cmaj.120876.

National Heart, Lung, and Blood Institute. "What Are Sleep Deprivation and Deficiency?" www.nhlbi.nih .gov/health/health-topics/topics/sdd/printall-index.html.

Additional Sources

www.health.harvard.edu/healthbeat/how-sleep-loss-threatens-your-health

https://sleepfoundation.org/media-center/press-release/annual-sleep-america-poll-exploring-connections -communications-technology-use-

www.sciencedaily.com/releases/2015/06/150615094255.htm

CHAPTER 1

Heffernan, Margaret. "Too Little Sleep: The New Performance Killer." CBSnews.com. www.cbsnews.com/ news/too-little-sleep-the-new-performance-killer/

Pomplun, Marc, Edward J. Silva, Joseph M. Ronda, Sean W. Cain, Mirjam Y. Münch, Charles A. Czeisler, and Jeanne F. Duffy. "The effects of circadian phase, time awake, and imposed sleep restriction on performing complex visual tasks: Evidence from comparative visual search." *Journal of Vision.* www.journalofvision .org/content/12/7/14.full

Taffinder, N. J., I. C. McManus, Y. Gul, R. C. G. Russell, and A. Darzi. "Effect of sleep deprivation on surgeons' dexterity on laparoscopy simulator." *The Lancet.* www.thelancet.com/pdfs/journals/lancet/ PIIS0140673698000348.pdf

Tracy, Abigail. "5 Tips to Get a Productive Night's Sleep." *Inc. Magazine* www.inc.com/abigail-tracy/five-tips -for-a-good-nights-sleep.html

Additional Sources

www.medicalnewstoday.com/articles/267611.php
http://articles.mercola.com/sites/articles/archive/2013/10/31/sleep-brain-detoxification.aspx
www.aasmnet.org/articles.aspx?id=4780
http://mountmessenger.msmc.edu/features/sleep-and-college-students/

CHAPTER 2

Brain Facts. "The Sleep-Wakefulness Cycle." www.brainfacts.org/sensing-thinking-behaving/sleep/articles/ 2012/the-sleep-wakefulness-cycle/

DiSalvo, David. "To Get More Sleep, Get More Sunlight." Forbes. www.forbes.com/sites/daviddisalvo/ 2013/06/18/to-get-more-sleep-get-more-sunlight/

Smart Tan. "Sun Exposure Leads to Better Sleep: Study" https://smarttan.com/news/index.php/sun-exposure-leads-to-better-sleep-study/

National Institute of Neurological Disorders and Stroke. "Brain Basics: Understanding Sleep." www.ninds.nih.gov/disorders/brain_basics/understanding_sleep.htm

University of Maryland Medical Center. "Melatonin." http://umm.edu/health/medical/altmed/supplement/melatonin

Wooten, M. D., D. Virgil. "How to Fall Asleep." http://health.howstuffworks.com/mental-health/sleep/basics/how-to-fall-asleep2.htm

Additional Sources

www.ncbi.nlm.nih.gov/pmc/articles/PMC297368/?page=4

www.womenshealthmag.com/life/boost-mood

www.menshealth.com/health/can-your-eyes-get-sunburned

www.globalspec.com/learnmore/optics_optical_components/optoelectronics/lux_meters_light_meters

www.ncbi.nlm.nih.gov/pmc/articles/PMC3779905/#B14

http://articles.mercola.com/sites/articles/archive/2012/03/26/maximizing-vitamin-d-exposure.aspx

www.ncbi.nlm.nih.gov/pmc/articles/PMC2077351/

www.psychologytoday.com/blog/prefrontal-nudity/201111/boosting-your-serotonin-activity

www.ncbi.nlm.nih.gov/pubmed/15677341

www.ncbi.nlm.nih.gov/pmc/articles/PMC3686562/

http://wellnessmama.com/24925/cortisol-myths/

www.ncbi.nlm.nih.gov/pubmed/22583560

http://blogs.webmd.com/sleep-disorders/2013/02/vitamin-d-deficiency-and-daytime-sleepiness.html

CHAPTER 3

Sutherland, Stephani. "Bright Screens Could Delay Bedtime." *Scientific American.* www.scientificamerican.com/article/bright-screens-could-delay-bedtime/

F.lux software. Research. http://justgetflux.com/research.html

Additional Sources

www.brighamandwomens.org/About_BWH/publicaffairs/news/PressReleases/PressRelease.aspx?sub=0&PageID=1962

http://blogs.scientificamerican.com/scicurious-brain/sleep-deprived-mind-your-dopamine/

http://news.stanford.edu/news/2001/march21/modafinil.html

www.psychologytoday.com/blog/brain-wise/201209/why-were-all-addicted-texts-twitter-and-google

CHAPTER 4

Breus, Dr. Michael. "New Details on Caffeine's Sleep-Disrupting Effects." Huffington Post. www.huffingtonpost.com/dr-michael-j-breus/caffeine-sleep_b_4454546.html

Paddock, PhD, Catharine. "Caffeine can disrupt sleep hours later." *Medical News Today.* www.medicalnewstoday.com/articles/268851.php

Purdy, Kevin. "What Caffeine Actually Does to Your Brain." *Life Hacker.* http://lifehacker.com/5585217/what-caffeine-actually-does-to-your-brain

Additional Sources

www.forbes.com/sites/travisbradberry/2012/08/21/caffeine-the-silent-killer-of-emotional-intelligence/

www.investorguide.com/article/11836/what-are-the-most-commonly-traded-commodities-igu/

www.foodinsight.org/CaffeineCreatedEqual#sthash.KZVwxWxx.dpbs

http://addictions.about.com/od/Caffeine/a/What-To-Expect-From-Caffeine-Withdrawal.htm

www.caffeineinformer.com/top-10-caffeine-health-benefits

http://blogs.scientificamerican.com/scicurious-brain/sleep-deprived-mind-your-dopamine/

www.brown.edu/Student_Services/Health_Services/Health_Education/nutrition_&_eating_concerns/caffeine.php

CHAPTER 5

Gradisar, M., L. Lack, H. Wright, J. Harris, and A. Brooks. "Do chronic primary insomniacs have impaired heat loss when attempting sleep?" www.ncbi.nlm.nih.gov/pubmed/16306160?ordinalpos=1&itool=Entrez System2.PEntrez.Pubmed.Pubmed_ResultsPanel.Pubmed_DefaultReportPanel.Pubmed_RVDocSum

Mercola, MD, Joseph. "Do Cold Temperatures Improve Sleep?" http://articles.mercola.com/sites/articles/archive/2009/12/19/Do-Cold-Temperatures-Improve-Sleep.aspx

O'Connor, Anahad. "The Claim: Cold Temperatures Improve Sleep." *The New York Times.* www.nytimes.com/2009/08/04/health/04real.html?_r=0

Additional Sources

http://time.com/3602415/sleep-problems-room-temperature/
http://healthland.time.com/2011/06/17/tip-for-insomniacs-cool-your-head-to-fall-asleep/
www.huffingtonpost.com/dr-christopher-winter/best-temperature-for-sleep_b_3705049.html
www.scientificamerican.com/article/putting-insomnia-on-ice/
www.chronobiology.ch/wp-content/uploads/publications/2006_07.pdf
www.silversurfers.com/health/foxys-fitness/oh-to-sleep/

CHAPTER 6

Chaudhary, MD, Kulreet. "Sleep and Longevity." www.doctoroz.com/blog/kulreet-chaudhary-md/sleep-and-longevity

Goel, Manisha. "What Is the Best Time to Go to Bed." *Life Hacker India* http://www.lifehacker.co.in/jugaad/What-Is-The-Best-Time-To-Go-To-Bed/articleshow/26421720.cms

Additional Sources

https://en.wikipedia.org/wiki/Neuroscience_of_sleep
www.fasebj.org/content/13/8/857.full
www.huffingtonpost.com/2014/08/14/shift-work-health-risks_n_5672965.html
www.huffingtonpost.com/2014/03/13/sleep-myths_n_4913209.html
www.theguardian.com/science/2015/jan/18/modern-world-bad-for-brain-daniel-j-levitin-organized-mind-information-overload
www.breastcancerfund.org/clear-science/radiation-chemicals-and-breast-cancer/light-at-night-and-melatonin.html
https://en.wikipedia.org/wiki/List_of_IARC_Group_2A_carcinogens
www.dnaindia.com/lifestyle/report-doctors-have-shorter-lifespan-than-patients-1341722
www.huffingtonpost.com/2012/07/21/police-sleep-shift-work-_n_1686727.html
www.ncbi.nlm.nih.gov/pubmed/12783938
www.ncbi.nlm.nih.gov/pubmed/16357603

CHAPTER 7

Clark, Ian. "The Perfect Mineral." http://store.activationproducts.com/magnesiuminfusion.html?AFFID=105206

Guise, Stephen. "50 Studies Suggest That Magnesium Deficiency Is Killing Us." Dumb Little Man: Tips for Life. www.dumblittleman.com/2013/08/50-studies-suggest-that-magnesium.html

Hyman, MD, Mark. "Magnesium: Meet the Most Powerful Relaxation Mineral Available." http://drhyman.com/blog/2010/05/20/magnesium-the-most-powerful-relaxation-mineral-available/

Nutrition Breakthroughs. "Insomnia: Studies Confirm Calcium and Magnesium Effective." Medical News Today. www.medicalnewstoday.com/releases/163169.php

Stevenson, Shawn. "Benefits of Magnesium" *The Shawn Stevenson Model.* http://theshawnstevensonmodel.com/benefits-of-magnesium/

Additional Sources

www.scientificamerican.com/article/gut-second-brain/
www.medicalnewstoday.com/articles/292693.php

http://news.sciencemag.org/biology/2014/10/are-your-bacteria-jet-lagged
http://articles.mercola.com/sites/articles/archive/2013/06/20/gut-brain-connection.aspx
www.ncbi.nlm.nih.gov/pubmed/22025877
www.ncbi.nlm.nih.gov/pubmed/18812627
www.ncbi.nlm.nih.gov/pubmed/22583560
www.ncbi.nlm.nih.gov/pubmed/22583560
http://blogs.webmd.com/sleep-disorders/2013/02/vitamin-d-deficiency-and-daytime-sleepiness.html
http://drgominak.com/vitamin-d-hormone.html
www.huffingtonpost.com/2013/08/01/nutrients-sleep_n_3671135.html -
http://womanitely.com/essential-nutrients-better-nights-sleep/5/
www.healthaliciousness.com/articles/foods-high-in-selenium.php
www.immunehealthscience.com/foods-with-melatonin.html
www.doctoroz.com/blog/susan-evans-md/parasites
www.mindbodygreen.com/0-11321/10-signs-you-may-have-a-parasite.html

CHAPTER 8

Hirshkowitz, PhD, Max, and Patricia B. Smith. *Sleep Disorders for Dummies.* http://books.google.com/books?id=r0PXwAzgrysC&pg=PT335&lpg=PT335&dq=running+water+effects+on+sleep&source=bl&ots=Az-SvlpiDB&sig=wkxBE5LK5CnKaQRdANF3hcRuEe0&hl=en&sa=X&ei=oXP6Uue3MsW8qgGXg4CQBw&ved=0CGMQ6AEwBw#v=onepage&q=running%20water%20effects%20on%20sleep&f=false

Huffington Post. "10 Best Houseplants to De-Stress Your Home and Purify the Air." www.huffingtonpost.com/2013/03/29/best-houseplants-destress_n_2964013.html

Merton, Amber. "Plant Therapy: How Plants Can Help You Sleep Better." *Plush Beds Blog.* www.plushbeds.com/blog/sleep-science/plant-therapy-how-plants-can-help-you-sleep-better/

Wheeling Jesuit University. "WJU Professor and Students Find Jasmine Odor Leads to More Restful Sleep, Decreased Anxiety, and Greater Mental Performance." www.wju.edu/about/adm_news_story.asp?iNewsID=539

Additional Sources

www.balancedbodyworkmassagetherapy.com/the-balanced-bodyworker-blog/lavender-essential-oil-for-sleep

CHAPTER 9

Bryn Mawr College. "Can Sex Cure Insomnia???" *Serendip.* http://serendip.brynmawr.edu/bb/neuro/neuro05/web2/contributor.html

Flash. "The 5 Health Benefits of Having an Orgasm." www.self.com/blogs/flash/2011/09/the-5-health-benefits-of-havin.html

Gloom. "Why Do Men Feel Sleepy After Sex?" *Mental Health Daily.* http://mentalhealthdaily.com/2013/04/24/why-do-men-feel-sleepy-after-sex-prolactin-oxytocin-vasopressin-et-al/

Jacques, Renee. "11 Reasons You Should Be Having More Orgasms." *Huffington Post.* www.huffingtonpost.com/2013/11/05/orgasm-health-benefits_n_4143213.html

Keeners, MD, Brigitte, Tillmann H.C. Kruger, MD, Stuart Brody, PhD, Sandra Schmidlin, Eva Naegeli, and Marcel Egli, PhD. "The Quality of Sexual Experience in Women Correlates with Post-Orgasmic Prolactin Surges: Results from an Experimental Prototype Study." *The Journal of Sexual Medicine.* www.ncbi.nlm.nih.gov/pubmed/23421490

Wenner, Melinda. "Why Do Guys Get Sleepy After Sex?" *Live Science.* www.livescience.com/32445-why-do-guys-get-sleepy-after-sex.html

Additional Sources

www.ncbi.nlm.nih.gov/pubmed/19570042
www.ncbi.nlm.nih.gov/pubmed/21890115
www.ncbi.nlm.nih.gov/pubmed/24435056
www.ncbi.nlm.nih.gov/pubmed/21699663
www.mensfitness.com/nutrition/sleep-or-die

https://sleepfoundation.org/sleep-news/possible-link-between-sleep-apnea-and-erectile-dysfunction

https://books.google.com/books?id=Kkts3AX9QVAC&pg=PA66&lpg=PA66&dq=orgasms+stress+study
&source=bl&ots=3f4uuHOU4j&sig=nYZccPCNut_Kn6Mp86n-pqBAVOI&hl=en&sa=X&ei=Fb5zU
vuFMorJsATg2oCABQ&ved=0CDoQ6AEwAQ#v=onepage&q=orgasms%20stress%20study&f=false

http://onlinelibrary.wiley.com/doi/10.1111/jsm.12858/pdf

www.psychologytoday.com/blog/dream-catcher/201108/oxytocin-sleep-and-dreams

www.ncbi.nlm.nih.gov/pubmed/23421490

https://en.wikipedia.org/wiki/Norepinephrine

www.ncbi.nlm.nih.gov/pmc/articles/PMC2812689/#R5

http://mentalhealthdaily.com/2013/04/24/why-do-men-feel-sleepy-after-sex-prolactin-oxytocin-vasopressin-et-al/

CHAPTER 10

Cass, MD, Hyla. "Let There Be Dark—and Melatonin." *Life Enhancement.* http://www.life-enhancement
.com/magazine/article/1677-let-there-be-dark-and-melatonin

Dvorsky, George. "Why we need to sleep in total darkness." *io9.* http://io9.com/why-we-need-to-sleep-in-total
-darkness-1497075228

Gooley, Joshua J., et al. "Exposure to Room Light before Bedtime Suppresses Melatonin Onset and Shortens
Melatonin Duration in Humans." *Journal of Clinical Endocrinology and Metabolism.* http://www.ncbi.nlm
.nih.gov/pmc/articles/PMC3047226/?report=classic

Pikul, Corrie. "How to Turn Your Bedroom into a Sleep Cave." *Huffington Post.* www.huffingtonpost
.com/2013/08/02/how-to-sleep-better-bedroom-tips_n_3673088.html

Stevenson, Shawn. "Help Me Sleep! 21 Ways to Cure Your Sleep Problems (Part 2)." *The Shawn Stevenson
Model.* http://theshawnstevensonmodel.com/21-cure-sleep-problem-pt2/

West, Kathleen E., et al. "Blue light from light-emitting diodes elicits a dose-dependent suppression of
melatonin in humans." Journal of Applied Physiology. http://jap.physiology.org/content/110/3/619.
abstract

Zukerman, Wendy. "Skin 'sees' the light to protect against sunshine." *New Scientist.* www.newscientist.com/
article/dn21127-skin-sees-the-light-to-protect-against-sunshine.html#.UvpkoXddUWw

Additional Sources

www.dianid.com/userfiles/editor/image/Color-temperature-in-Kelvin(1).jpg

Book: Lights Out by T.S. Wiley with Bent Formby, Ph.D.—Chapter 5—Section: Sleeping, Dreaming, & Dying

www.brighamandwomens.org/about_bwh/publicaffairs/news/pressreleases/PressRelease.aspx?sub=0&
PageID=1962

www.huffingtonpost.com/2014/12/23/reading-before-bed_n_6372828.html

www.ncbi.nlm.nih.gov/pubmed/21552190

http://products.mercola.com/himalayan-salt/himalayan-salt-lamps.htm

www.health.harvard.edu/staying-healthy/blue-light-has-a-dark-side

CHAPTER 11

Appalachian State University. "Early morning exercise is best for reducing blood pressure and improving sleep."
www.news.appstate.edu/2011/06/13/early-morning-exercise/

Davis, Jeanie Lerche. "Morning Exercise May Help You Sleep." WebMD. www.webmd.com/menopause/
news/20031104/morning-exercise-may-help-you-sleep

Experience Life. "Exercise Early, Sleep Better. http://experiencelife.com/newsflashes/exercise-early-sleep
-deep/

Stevenson, Shawn. "Fatal Fat Loss Mistake#3—Working Out At Night." *The Shawn Stevenson Model.*
http://theshawnstevensonmodel.com/fat-loss-mistake-working-out-at-night/

Widrich, Leo. "What Happens to Our Brains When We Exercise and How It Makes Us Happier."
Buffer. http://blog.bufferapp.com/why-exercising-makes-us-happier?utm_content=bufferd1a95&utm
_medium=social&utm_source=twitter.com&utm_campaign=buffer

Wooten, MD, Virgil D. "How to Fall Asleep." *How Stuff Works.* http://health.howstuffworks.com/mental
-health/sleep/basics/how-to-fall-asleep1.htm

Additional Sources

http://guides.library.unk.edu/content.php?pid=432580&sid=3538852

https://escholarship.org/uc/item/385578q5

www.ncbi.nlm.nih.gov/pubmed/23946713

www.journalsleep.org/ViewAbstract.aspx?pid=28194

www.huffingtonpost.com/dr-michael-j-breus/sleep-athletic-performance_b_901615.html

www.huffingtonpost.com/dr-michael-j-breus/sports-sleep_b_2160565.html

www.fatiguescience.com/blog/infographic-why-athletes-should-make-sleep-a-priority-in-their-daily-training

www.ncbi.nlm.nih.gov/pmc/articles/PMC2883039/?tool=pubmed

www.ncbi.nlm.nih.gov/pubmed/21550729

www.ncbi.nlm.nih.gov/pubmed/23946713

www.edinformatics.com/news/exercise_and_aging.htm

CHAPTER 12

Becker, Joshua. "18 Good Reasons to Get the TV Out of Your Bedroom." *Becoming Minimalist*. www.becomingminimalist.com/18-darn-good-reasons-to-get-the-tv-out-of-the-bedroom/

Gilbert, Jason. "Smartphone Addiction: Staggering Percentage of Humans Couldn't Go One Day Without Their Phone." Huffington Post. www.huffingtonpost.com/2012/08/16/smartphone-addiction-time-survey_n_1791790.html

Gittleman, Ann Louise. "Hormones, Cell Phones, and EMFs." *Are You Zapped*. www.areyouzapped.com/articles/83

Lean, Geoffrey. "Mobile phone radiation wrecks your sleep." *The Independent*. http://www.independent.co.uk/life-style/health-and-families/health-news/mobile-phone-radiation-wrecks-your-sleep-771262.html

Mercola, MD, Joseph. "NEW Urgent Warning to All Cell Phone Users." http://articles.mercola.com/sites/articles/archive/2012/06/16/emf-safety-tips.aspx

_____. "Cell Phones Raise Children's Risk of Brain Cancer 500 Percent." http://articles.mercola.com/sites/articles/archive/2008/10/11/cell-phones-raise-children-s-risk-of-brain-cancer-500-percent.aspx

Macrae, Fiona. "Computer in your child's bedroom disturbs sleep and can lead to memory problems and poor marks in school." *Daily Mail*. www.dailymail.co.uk/health/article-2378417/Computer-childs-bedroom-disturbs-sleep-lead-memory-problems-poor-marks-school.html

National Cancer Institute. "Magnetic Field Exposure and Cancer: Questions and Answers." www.cancer.gov/cancertopics/factsheet/Risk/magnetic-fields

Parker-Pope, Tara. "A One-Eyed Invader in the Bedroom." *The New York Times*. www.nytimes.com/2008/03/04/health/04well.html?_r=0

Talreja, Prerna. "Sleeping with Your Phone Is Bad for Your Health—Obviously." *Policy Mic*. www.policymic.com/articles/31199/sleeping-with-your-phone-is-bad-for-your-health-obviously

Riggs, Roy." The Little-Known Dangers of EMFs and How to Protect You and Your Family." *Body Ecology*. http://bodyecology.com/articles/little-known-dangers-of-emf.php#.UxSwdfRdUWx

Additional Sources

www.ncbi.nlm.nih.gov/pubmed/24772943

www.electricsense.com/988/where-is-the-place-you-absolutely-must-start-if-you-want-to-protect-yourself-from-electromagnetic-radiation/#sthash.Icnnq4sR.dpuf

www.ncbi.nlm.nih.gov/pubmed/23479077

www.ncbi.nlm.nih.gov/pubmed/17548154

www.scientificamerican.com/article/mind-control-by-cell/

www.electricsense.com/3544/wifi-radiation-how-to-protect-yourself/

www.ncbi.nlm.nih.gov/pubmed/22112647

www.medicineonline.com/news/12/3081/TV-in-the-bedroom-halves-your-sex-life-study.html

CHAPTER 13

Brandt, Michelle L. "Researchers ID best hours to sleep when time is limited: People who rest in the early morning do better than those who sleep late at night." *Stanford Report*. http://news.stanford.edu/news/2003/may28/sleep.html

Dean, MD, Carolyn. "Magnesium—The Weight Loss Cure." *Natural News.* www.naturalnews.com/036049 _magnesium_weight_loss_cure.html

Gregoire, Carolyn. "Being Overweight, Obese Linked to Release of Stress Hormone Cortisol After Eating." *Huffington Post.* www.huffingtonpost.com/2013/06/20/stress-weight-gain_n_3459755.html

Gunnars, Kris. "23 Studies on Low-Carb and Low-Fat Diets—Time to Retire the Fad." *Authority Nutrition.* http://authoritynutrition.com/23-studies-on-low-carb-and-low-fat-diets/

National Sleep Foundation. "Obesity and Sleep." www.sleepfoundation.org/sleep-topics/obesity-and-sleep/ page/0%2C1/

MacGill, Markus. "Obesity link to lack of sleep suggested by brain scans." *Medical News Today.* www .medicalnewstoday.com/articles/264539.php

Pessoney, Stacy A. "Basic Magnesium Deficiency Causes Obesity and Diabetes." *Wholesale Nutrition.* http://nutri.com/blog/2014/02/basic-magnesium-deficiency-causes-obesity-and-diabetes/

Shafii, Mohammad, Duncan R. Macmillan, Mary P. Key, Nancy Kaufman, and Irwin D. Nahinsky. "Case Study: Melatonin in Severe Obesity." *Journal of the American Academy of Child and Adolescent Psychiatry.* http://www.sciencedirect.com/science/article/pii/S0890856709664467

Additional Sources

www.huffingtonpost.com/2012/04/11/shift-work-sleep-type-2-diabetes-obesity_n_1418394.html

http://easyhealthoptions.com/best-foods-for-a-good-nights-sleep/

http://healthland.time.com/2012/11/06/cant-sleep-losing-belly-fat-might-help/

www.health.harvard.edu/blog/losing-weight-and-belly-fat-improves-sleep-201211145531

http://sleepdisorders.about.com/od/sleepandgeneralhealth/a/How-Does-Being-Overweight-Affect-Your -Sleep.htm

CHAPTER 14

Arnedt, J. T., D. J. Rohsenow, A. B. Almeida, S. K. Hunt, M. Gokhale, D. J. Gottlieb, and J. Howland,. "Sleep following alcohol intoxication in healthy, young adults: effects of sex and family history of alcoholism." *Alcoholism: Clinical and Experimental Research.* www.ncbi.nlm.nih.gov/pubmed/21323679

Park, Alice. "Can't Sleep? It May Be Affecting Your Memory." *Time.* http://healthland.time.com/2012/02/16/ cant-sleep-it-may-be-affecting-your-memory/

Ross, Valerie. "Alcohol Side Effects: 4 Ways Drinking Messes with Your Sleep." *Huffington Post.* www.huffingtonpost.com/2013/05/17/alcohol-side-effects-drinking-sleep_n_3286434.html

Goins, Liesa. "How to Hold Your Liquor." WebMD. www.webmd.com/balance/features/how-to-hold-your -liquor

Wikipedia. "Sleep and memory." http://en.wikipedia.org/wiki/Sleep_and_memory

Rosenberg, PhD, Russell. "How Alcohol Can Ruin Your Sleep." *Huffington Post.* www.huffingtonpost.com/ russell-rosenberg-phd/alcohol-sleep_b_902578.html

Additional Sources

http://thechart.blogs.cnn.com/2011/11/09/driving-drowsy-as-dangerous-as-driving-drunk-studies-show/

www.discovery.com/tv-shows/mythbusters/about-this-show/tired-vs-drunk-driving/

www.webmd.com/sleep-disorders/news/20130118/alcohol-sleep

www.ayureka.com/wp-content/uploads/2014/02/Alcohol-Sleep-Chart4a.jpg

www.jneurosci.org/content/34/23/7733.full

www.livescience.com/12870-guys-gals-drunk-sleep-science.html

CHAPTER 15

Breene, Sophia. "The Best (and Worse) Positions for Sleeping." *Greatist.* http://greatist.com/happiness/ best-sleep-positions

BuzzFeed. "What Your Sleeping Position Says About You." https://www.youtube.com/watch?v=XjoqsIgJTk0

Dale, Heather. "The Pros and Cons of Sleeping on Your Side, Back, and Stomach. *PopSugar.* www.fitsugar .com/Which-Sleep-Position-Healthiest-14571804

Hit Full. "22 Funny-Awkward Sleeping Positions." www.hitfull.com/pictures/pset.php?set=funny_crazy _Awkward_Sleeping_positions

Pratiks. "3 Positions for 2 People Sleeping Together." www.youtube.com/watch?v=rcV1CGN3tvA

Search Results: Sleep Position. YouTube.com www.youtube.com/results?search_query=sleep%20position&sm=3

UNP. *Sleeping Style Chart.* www.unp.me/f8/whts-your-sleeping-style-215474/

Wikipedia. "Snoring." http://en.wikipedia.org/wiki/Snoring

Vojta, Prof. Václav. "Who Developed Vojta Diagnostics and Therapy?" *The Vojta Principle.* http://vojtakonzept.de/index.php?option=com_content&view=article&id=47&Itemid=7&lang=en

Frew, David R. "Transcendental Meditation and Productivity." *Academy of Management Journal.* http://amj.aom.org/content/17/2/362.short

Additional Sources

www.ncbi.nlm.nih.gov/pmc/articles/PMC2549463/

www.healthychild.com/has-the-cause-of-crib-death-sids-been-found/

www.healthychild.com/are-toxic-gases-in-crib-mattresses-causing-crib-death-sids/

CHAPTER 16

American Academy of Sleep Medicine. "Meditation May Be an Effective Treatment for Insomnia." Science Daily. http://www.sciencedaily.com/releases/2009/06/090609072719.htm

"Better Sleep Through Meditation: 4 Techniques to Try Tonight." *Health Magazine.* www.health.com/health/condition-article/0,,20189101,00.html

Finerminds. "Meet Your Brain Waves—Introducing Alpha, Beta, Theta, Delta, and Gamma." www.finerminds.com/mind-power/brain-waves/

Meditations Mind Matters. "Brainwaves." www.meditations-uk.com/information/brain_waves.html

Trafton, Anne. "The benefits of meditation." *MIT News.* http://web.mit.edu/newsoffice/2011/meditation-0505.html

Additional Sources

http://hpq.sagepub.com/content/14/1/60.short

www.ncbi.nlm.nih.gov/pubmed/25233147

www.health.harvard.edu/staying-healthy/the-health-benefits-of-tai-chi

www.ncbi.nlm.nih.gov/pubmed/15707256

www.huffingtonpost.com/elaine-gavalas/yoga-sleep_b_1719825.html

http://what-when-how.com/wp-content/uploads/2012/04/tmp3626.jpg

www.collective-evolution.com/2014/10/02/your-ancestors-didnt-sleep-like-you-are-were-doing-it-wrong/

CHAPTER 17

Asprey, Dave. "Sleep Hacking Part 3`` Falling Asleep Fast with Biochemistry." *Bulletproof: The State of High Performance.* www.bulletproofexec.com/sleep-hacking-part-3-falling-asleep-fast-with-biochemistry/

Ehrlich, NMD, Steven D. "5-Hydroxytryptophan (5-HTP)." University Of Maryland Medical Reference Guide. http://umm.edu/health/medical/altmed/supplement/5hydroxytryptophan-5htp

_____. "Kava kava." University Of Maryland Medical Reference Guide http://umm.edu/health/medical/altmed/herb/kava-kava

_____. "Valerian." University Of Maryland Medical Reference Guide https://umm.edu/health/medical/altmed/herb/valerian

Smucker, MPH, PhD, Celeste M. "Chamomile helps with anxiety, sleeplessness and depression." Natural News. www.naturalnews.com/034454_chamomile_anxiety_depression.html

Sisson, Mark. "Why Melatonin Is a Dangerous Supplement." *Mark's Daily Apple.* www.marksdailyapple.com/before-you-close-your-eyes-make-sure-theyre-open/#axzz2vD0hbsog

Srivastava, Janmejai K., Eswar Shankar, and Sanjay Gupta. "Chamomile: A herbal medicine of the past with a bright future (Review)." *Molecular Medicine Reports.* www.spandidos-publications.com/mmr/3/6/895

Additional Sources

http://examine.com/supplements/apigenin/

www.ncbi.nlm.nih.gov/pmc/articles/PMC2995283/#R47

www.ncbi.nlm.nih.gov/pubmed/20306120
www.ncbi.nlm.nih.gov/pubmed/17143534
www.ncbi.nlm.nih.gov/pubmed/15181652
www.doctoroz.com/episode/why-melatonin-may-be-dangerous-your-sleep
www.ncbi.nlm.nih.gov/pubmed/9406047

CHAPTER 18

Agliata, Kate. "Characteristics of Nocturnal Animals." *eHow*. www.ehow.com/info_8742878_characteristics-nocturnal-animals.html

Gonzalez, Robert T. "Why is it so impossible to get out of bed in the morning?" *io9*. http://io9.com/why-is-it-so-impossible-to-get-out-of-bed-in-the-morning-1348209324

Mercola, MD, Joseph. "Why You Should Never Sleep with TV or Dim Lights On..." http://articles.mercola.com/sites/articles/archive/2011/02/19/why-you-should-never-sleep-with-tv-or-dim-lights-on.aspx

Rettner, Rachel. "Avoiding Depression: Sleeping in Dark Room May Help." *Live Science*. www.livescience.com/9004-avoiding-depression-sleeping-dark-room.html?utm_source=feedburner&utm_medium=feed&utm_campaign=Feed%3A+livescience%2Fhealthscitech+%28LiveScience.com+Health+Sci Tech%29

Williams, Ray B. "Early Risers Are Happier, Healthier, and More Productive Than Night Owls." *Psychology Today*. www.psychologytoday.com/blog/wired-success/201208/early-risers-are-happier-healthier-and-more-productive-night-owls

Marks, MD, Tracey. "How to Become a Morning Person." *Huffington Post*. www.huffingtonpost.com/tracey-marks-md/morning-person_b_864377.html

Goudreau, Jenna. "10 Advantages of Waking Up Early." *Forbes Woman*. http://shine.yahoo.com/healthy-living/10-advantages-waking-early-195900205.html

Babauta, Leo. "The Most Successful Techniques for Rising Early." *Zen Habits*. http://zenhabits.net/early/

CHAPTER 19

Additional resources

www.sleepreviewmag.com/2014/05/massage-therapy-sleep/
www.ncbi.nlm.nih.gov/pmc/articles/PMC3018656/
www.massagetherapy.com/articles/index.php/article_id/911/Moderate-vs-Light-Pressure-in-Massage
https://en.wikipedia.org/wiki/Massage
www.ncbi.nlm.nih.gov/pubmed/19034252
www.ncbi.nlm.nih.gov/pubmed/19034253
www.everydayhealth.com/sleep/insomnia/tips/guide-to-relaxation.aspx
www.oprah.com/health/The-Health-Benefits-of-Massage
http://news.emory.edu/stories/2012/08/rapaport_frequent_massage/campus.html

CHAPTER 20

Gates, Sara. "Do Women Need Bras? French Study Says Brassieres Are a 'False Necessity'." *Huffington Post*. www.huffingtonpost.com/2013/04/11/women-bras-study-france-false-necessity_n_3062114.html

Ghana News. "Why Sleeping Without Clothes Is Good." www.spyghana.com/why-sleeping-without-clothes-is-good/

Krempf, Antoine. "Breasts would be better without a bra." *France Info*. www.franceinfo.fr/societe/les-seins-se-portent-mieux-sans-soutien-gorge-947307-2013-04-10

Low-Blue-Light Glasses. www.lowbluelights.com

Singer, Sydney Ross. "Droop Phobia, the Bra, and Breast Cancer." *Killer Culture*. http://www.killerculture.com/droop-phobia-the-bra-and-breast-cancer/

Stevenson, Shawn. "Dressed to Kill—The Dangers of Wearing Bras and Constrictive Clothing with Medical Anthropologist Sydney Singer." http://theshawnstevensonmodel.com/dangers-wearing-bras/

Additional Sources

https://en.wikipedia.org/wiki/Cremaster_muscle
www.medicalnewstoday.com/articles/247826.php
www.ncbi.nlm.nih.gov/pubmed/2136041

CHAPTER 21

Chevalier, G., S. T. Sinatra, J. L. Oschman, and R. M. Delany. "Earthing (grounding) the human body reduces blood viscosity—a major factor in cardiovascular disease." *Journal of Alternative and Complementary Medicine*. www.ncbi.nlm.nih.gov/pubmed/22757749

Ghaly, MD, Maurice, and Dale Teplitx, MA. "The Biologic Effects of Grounding the Human Body During Sleep as Measured by Cortisol Levels and Subjective Reporting of Sleep, Pain, and Stress." *Journal of Alternative and Complementary Medicine*. www.ncbi.nlm.nih.gov/pubmed/15650465

Kiefer, Dale. "Superoxide Dismutase Boosting the Body's Primary Antioxidant Defense." Life Etension Magazine. www.lef.org/magazine/mag2006/jun2006_report_sod_01.htm

The Earthing Institute. "Are you grounded in water—the ocean, a lake, your swimming pool, your bathtub?" http://earthinginstitute.net/qa/%E2%97%8F-are-you-grounded-in-water-the-ocean-a-lake-your-swimming-pool-your-bathtub/

Additional Sources

www.medicalnewstoday.com/articles/207877.php
www.ncbi.nlm.nih.gov/pmc/articles/PMC3265077/

14-DAY SLEEP MAKEOVER

Lynn, Aaron. "Evening Rituals: Getting Better Sleep with a Little Preparation." *Asian Efficiency*. www.asianefficiency.com/health/evening-rituals-getting-better-sleep-with-a-little-preparation/

Griffel, Mattan. "Unconscious Incompetence and the Four Stages of Learning." *Medium*. https://medium.com/self-investment/ad5583abf646

Tartakovsky, MS, Margarita. "12 Ways to Shut Off Your Brain Before Bedtime." *Psych Central*. http://psychcentral.com/lib/12-ways-to-shut-off-your-brain-before-bedtime/0006577

INDEX